Medical Examination Made Memorable (MEMM)

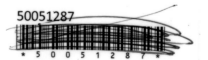

50051287

Medical Examination Made Memorable (MEMM)

SHAHED YOUSAF

GP Trainee
West Midlands

WITHDRAWN
THE LIBRARY OF
TRINITY COLLEGE DUBLIN

AUTHORISED: KM

DATE: 22-11-22

Radcliffe Publishing
Oxford • New York

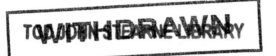

Radcliffe Publishing Ltd
18 Marcham Road
Abingdon
Oxon OX14 1AA
United Kingdom

S7
610.7
R03;1

www.radcliffe-oxford.com
Electronic catalogue and worldwide online ordering facility.

© 2010 Shahed Yousaf
Illustrations © 2010 Shahed Yousaf

Shahed Yousaf has asserted his right under the Copyright, Designs and Patents Act 1998 to be identified as the author of this work.

All rights reserved. No part of this publication may be reproduced, stored in a retrieval system or transmitted, in any form or by any means, electronic, mechanical, photocopying, recording or otherwise, without the prior permission of the copyright owner.

British Library Cataloguing in Publication Data
A catalogue record for this book is available from the British Library.

ISBN-13: 978 184619 060 5

The paper used for the text pages of this book
is FSC certified. FSC (The Forest Stewardship
Council) is an international network to promote
responsible management of the world's forests.

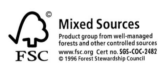

Mixed Sources
Product group from well-managed
forests and other controlled sources
www.fsc.org Cert no. SGS-COC-2482
© 1996 Forest Stewardship Council

Typeset by Pindar NZ, Auckland, New Zealand
Printed and bound by TJI Digital, Padstow, Cornwall, UK

Contents

Preface

What is memory?

A dictionary definition would be 'the ability to recall past information or experience'. It is beyond the remit of this book to grapple with the complexities of different types of memories and where they are stored in the brain. Instead, it is more practical to ask what makes something memorable, and how we can utilise this to aid learning and remembering.

In order for something to be memorable it has to fulfil two criteria. It has to be significant information – and therefore naturally committed to memory – and it has to be accessible or it will be forgotten. There are various psychological theories about how remembering occurs. The psychologist Frederic Bartlett states that we remember things based on what we already know, and create a context for new information, like a web. Cognitive processing models suggest that different individuals prefer information to be presented in different ways. One of these models is the VARK system which utilises a questionnaire to identify the modes of information people prefer to process Visual, Aural, Reading and Writing, Kinaesthetic and Multi-modal.

Information is best recalled if it makes a link with something already known and therefore we have mentioned well-known people who have various health conditions. We have carefully produced images, some of which are caricatures and knowingly bizarre, to act as a cue to recall the information. The information itself is broken down into easily recallable chunks, so as not to overwhelm. We have used mnemonics only where they add something unique, because not everybody finds them useful.

Information is best recalled if it is discussed with others in order to stimulate the aural component of memory and to introduce a narrative to the memory. Practising physical skills leads to kinaesthetic memorisation – muscle memory. Most importantly we have attempted to make the information fun and enjoyable to learn. The easier it is to learn, the easier it is to recall. Happy learning and remembering!

Shahed Yousaf
January 2010

About the author

Dr Shahed Yousaf graduated from Warwick Medical School in 2006. He is the co-author of *Mnemonics for Medical Undergraduates*, which was published in his final year at medical school by PasTest books. Shahed is now a GP trainee in the West Midlands. He maintains an interest in writing, illustrating and medical education.

Contributor
Mubeen Chaudhry
Radiology Trainee

Acknowledgements

Passing on medical knowledge is a duty incumbent upon all medical health professionals and we would like to take this opportunity to thank, in particular, the following people who have aided our understanding of various aspects of medicine:

Amdad Ahmed, Sameen Akhtar, Imran Arshad, Irfan Babar, Nisha Gohil, Pasi Guti, Sadat Edroos, Rebekah Mansfield, Asam Murtaza, Vinod Patel, Mohammed Saeed, Matthew Sommerlad, Suleiman Sultan.

I would like to thank Mohammed Yousaf, Bilqees Begum and Shahzadi Yousaf.

Introduction

Ethics
Hippocratic Oath
The Hippocratic Oath is taken by doctors swearing to practise medicine ethically. It is attributed to Hippocrates, the father of western medicine, in the 4th century BC. The second paragraph states the obligation to pass on medical knowledge. There are various modern versions of the Hippocratic Oath but all draw on common ethical principles.

The original Hippocratic Oath (translated from Greek)

I swear by Apollo, the healer, Asclepius, Hygieia, and Panacea, and I take to witness all the gods, all the goddesses, to keep according to my ability and my judgment, the following Oath and agreement:

To consider dear to me, as my parents, him who taught me this art; to live in common with him and, if necessary, to share my goods with him; To look upon his children as my own brothers, to teach them this art.

I will prescribe regimens for the good of my patients according to my ability and my judgment and never do harm to anyone.

I will not give a lethal drug to anyone if I am asked, nor will I advise such a plan; and similarly I will not give a woman a pessary to cause an abortion.

But I will preserve the purity of my life and my arts.

I will not cut for stone, even for patients in whom the disease is manifest; I will leave this operation to be performed by practitioners, specialists in this art.

In every house where I come I will enter only for the good of my patients, keeping myself far from all intentional ill-doing and all seduction and especially from the pleasures of love with women or with men, be they free or slaves.

All that may come to my knowledge in the exercise of my profession or in daily commerce with men, which ought not to be spread abroad, I will keep secret and will never reveal.

If I keep this oath faithfully, may I enjoy my life and practise my art, respected by all men and in all times; but if I swerve from it or violate it, may the reverse be my lot.

Common ethical principles in medicine (BANJ)
B Beneficence (doing good) – arguably, the most important principle.
A Autonomy (self-determination).
N Non-maleficence (do no harm).
J Justice (equality for all).

The Geneva Convention (1948)
The Geneva Convention is a revision of the Hippocratic Oath and was designed to reaffirm the ethics of the medical profession in the aftermath of the Nuremberg trials in which several physicians were prosecuted.

> *At the time of being admitted as a member of the medical professions:*
> *I solemnly pledge myself to consecrate my life to the service of humanity*
> *I will practise my profession with conscience and dignity;*
> *I will give to my teachers the respect and gratitude which is their due;*
> *The health and life of my patient will be my first consideration;*
> *I will respect the secrets which are confided in me;*
> *I will maintain, by all means in my power, the honour and the noble traditions of the medical profession;*
> *My colleagues will be my brothers;*
> *I will not permit considerations of religion, nationality, race, party politics, or social standing to intervene between my duty and my patient;*
> *I will maintain the utmost respect for human life from the time of its conception; even under threat, I will not use my medical knowledge contrary to the laws of humanity;*
> *I make these promises solemnly, freely and upon my honour.*

The Declaration of Helsinki
The Declaration of Helsinki (6th revision, 2008) is a set of ethical principles regarding human experimentation and research developed by the World Medical Association (WMA). The fundamental principles are respect for the individual (Article 8), their right to self-determination, and their right to make informed decisions (Articles 20, 21 and 22) regarding participation in research, both initially and during the course of the research.

Equipment
Be in the habit of carrying around with you at least a stethoscope, pen-torch and alcohol gel as well as your identity badge. You should have access to the following equipment on the ward:
- alcohol gel, hot running water and soap
- auroscope
- cotton wool balls
- disposable gloves
- measuring tape

- ophthalmoscope
- otoscope
- patella hammer
- pen-torch
- sphygmomanometer
- stethoscope
- tendon hammer
- tongue depressors
- tuning fork

General history and examination

Contents
- Three phases of clinical examination
- Safe approach to a patient
- Medical history: presenting complaint, history of presenting complaint, pain history, past medical history, risk factors, medications/allergies, family history, social history, general enquiries, functional enquiry
- Physical examination: pre-examination checklist, inspection, speech, dehydration, nutritional status, body odour, facial appearance, hair, lymph nodes, hands
- Abbreviated mental test
- Breast examination
- Clubbing
- Nails
- Skin colour
- Thyroid examination

Three phases of clinical examination (HEP)
H History taking
E Examination and impression
P Plan

SAFE approach to a patient
Before approaching a patient ensure **SAFE**:
S Setting – adequate privacy such as a room, if examining at the bedside draw the curtains and use a quiet voice especially with sensitive topics.
A Appearance – identity badge, appropriate clothes, clean hands and nails
F Facts about the case – not all patients know their full diagnosis, do not say anything inappropriate or unethical. Do not give false hope.

E Equipment – *see* Equipment list, p. x.

Medical history

State the following before beginning any history:
- Introduction
- Permission
- How long it will take
- Confidential
- History followed by examination
- Name
- DoB
- Age

* Date and time need to be documented

Presenting complaint

'Can you tell me when you were last well and in your own words, what has happened since then?'

(Do not interrupt the patient as they talk for at least 2–3 minutes, provide appropriate non-verbal cues and show them that you are paying attention.)

History of presenting complaint

- 'So you have told me about your illness; can I ask you if you think there was anything that might have **TRIGGERED** the onset of your illness?
- And what has been the **COURSE** of your illness – has it got **better over time, worse over time**, or has it **stayed the same**?
- Have there been any periods where you have been **completely free** of the problem?
- Over the course of **24 hrs** when are you most bothered by your complaint?'

To recall this the mnemonic **OPERATES** may help:
O **O**nset of complaint
P **P**rogress of complaint
E **E**xacerbating factors
R **R**elieving factors
A **A**ssociated symptoms
T **T**iming
E **E**pisodes of being symptom free
S Relevant **S**ystemic and general enquiry can be added here

Pain history

A pain history can follow a similar format as shown below **LOTTRAADIO:**
L **L**ocation
O **O**nset – what were you doing when it started?
T **T**iming – how long did it last?

T Type (sharp/throbbing/gnawing)
R Radiation
A Associated symptoms (nausea/vomiting/sweating)
A Aggravating factors
D Decreasing factors
I Intensity on a scale of 1–10 with 10 being the worst pain imaginable
O Offset – what were you doing when it stopped?

Alternatively, **SOCRATIC:**
S Site
O Onset – what were you doing when it started?
C Character (sharp/throbbing/gnawing)
R Radiation
A Associated symptoms (nausea/vomiting/sweating)
T Timing – how long did it last?
I Improving/worsening factors
C Count the pain on a scale of 1–10 with 10 being the worst pain imaginable

Past medical history
- Hospital admissions
- Illnesses (*see* MCJ THHREADS below)
- Operations
- Immunisation status
- Overseas travel

Risk factors
Most apt for atheromatous disease, mnemonic – **SHAHED** (the author of this book)
S Smoking
H Hypertension
A Alcohol
H Hyperlipidaemia
E Exercise and healthy Eating
D DM

MCJ THHREADS
M MI
C Cancer
J Jaundice
T TB
H Hypertension
H Hypercholesterolaemia
R Rheumatic fever as a child
E Epilepsy

A Asthma
D DM
S Stroke

Medications/allergies (PILLS)
P Pills patient is taking
I Injections, e.g. Insulin/Inhalers (as some patients forget to mention when asked about their medications)
LL ILLicit drug use
S Sensitivities to anything, i.e. allergies, what was the reaction?

Family history
- Are your **parents** still with us?
- If not, what did they pass away from?
- Do you have any **siblings** with the same illness?
- Have any of your siblings passed away?
- Do you have **children**, do they have anything similar?

Social history (SAADLES)
S Smoking – pack years? 20/day for 1 year = 1 pack year
A Alcohol consumption in units? 1 unit = ½ pint beer/1 glass wine/1 measure spirit (female 14 units = 7 pints lager/male 21 units = 10½ pints lager)
ADL Activities of Daily Living – how do you manage with bathing, cooking, cleaning, shopping? This section should also incorporate what **job** the person does and whether their illness could be related to this.
E Enjoyment activities, i.e. recreational activities/hobbies
S Social support, i.e. family, neighbours, carers, GP home visits, district nurses, home help, meals on wheels and financial problems.

In a respiratory history, it is important to include the following points **SOD PETe**
S Smoking
O Occupational exposure to various metals, allergens, etc.
D Drugs being used – some medications cause pulmonary fibrosis, e.g. amiodarone
PET PET exposure, e.g. cats, pigeons, etc.

General enquiries
In every history don't forget to ask about the **4 (FAWR)** non-specific symptoms the patient may exhibit:
F Fever
A Appetite
W Weight loss (unintentional)
R Reduced energy, i.e. fatigue/lethargy

Functional enquiry

Neurology

- Auditory problems
- Double vision/dizziness or problems with balance/ coordination
- Epilepsy enquiry
- Faints
- Hallucinations
- Headaches
- Intention/resting tremor
- Muscles feel weak
- Numbness
- Speech problems
- Sphincter disturbance; urinary/bowel
- Syncope
- Tingling sensation – pins and needles

Cardiology

- Angina pectoris, i.e. chest pain
- Heart beat awareness, i.e. palpitations
- Oedema – ankle swelling, gravity-dependent areas
- Rheumatic fever as a child
- Shortness of breath
- Syncope
- Tiredness

Respiratory

- Chest pain, pleuritic
- Cough, non-productive, productive – sputum colour, quantity
- Haemoptysis
- Shortness of breath
- Feeling weak, i.e. lethargy
- Fever
- Funny noises on breathing, i.e. wheeze and stridor
- Speech impaired, i.e. hoarseness

Gastroenterology

Consider anatomically from entry to exit

Mouth

- Do you have trouble with your teeth?
- Do you have any difficulty chewing your food?
- Do you have difficulty swallowing your food?

Pharynx and oesophagus
- Difficulty in swallowing (dysphagia)
- Pain on swallowing (odynophagia)
- Do you have heartburn?

Stomach
- Any nausea or vomiting?
- Is there anything unusual in the vomitus such as bile, blood (haematemesis)?
- Do you have ulcers, relieved or exacerbated by food?

Liver, biliary tract and pancreas
- Abdominal swelling – ascites
- Alcohol consumption
- Chills, i.e. fever and rigors
- Colic, i.e. right upper quadrant
- Confusion and drowsiness; hepatic encephalopathy
- Gynaecomastia
- Hepatitis enquiry, i.e. been abroad recently, in contact with anyone suffering from this, IV drug use, unprotected sex/anal sex
- Impaired glucose tolerance due to decreased pancreatic function hence polyuria, polydipsia and weight loss; DM?
- Jaundice
- Petechiae, i.e. easy bruising and bleeding

Small and large bowels
- Constipation
- Diarrhoea
- Stools – dark stools, melaena (tarry, foul-smelling), mucus, pale.
- Pain on passing stools
- Piles – fresh blood on toilet paper

Renal system (FUN PHISS)
F Increased Frequency of urination
U Urgency
N Nocturia
P Polyuria
H Hesitancy
I Incontinence, urinary/Incomplete emptying of bladder
S Stinging on urination?
S Something unusual in the urine, blood? discolouration? 'frothy'?

Musculoskeletal (STABS)

S Stiffness: morning or evening?
T Tenderness or pain in muscles or joints?
A Affected joints distribution, i.e. symmetrical, axial or peripheral?
B Bruising or bleeding into joint?
S Swellings around joint?

Psychological state (SAD CASE)

S Suicidal ideations
A Anxiety
D Decreased mood/Delusions/Disordered thought
C Difficulty Concentrating
A Auditory or other hallucinations?
S Difficulties Sleeping
E Eating normally?

During the course of the history taking, if you suspect that the patient is confused, quantify confusion by doing a bedside abbreviated Mental state examination. *See* Abbreviated Mental state examination, p. 67.

Physical examination

Pre-examination checklist (WIPERS)

W Wash your hands.
I Introduce yourself to the patient with a handshake and note its characteristics; show identification if required.
P Ask Permission to take a history and examine; Position the patient, supine on a couch raised at 45 degrees, apart from a gastrointestinal examination, where the patient lies flat.
E Expose the area to be examined but preserve the patient's dignity (male examiners require a female chaperone); Enquire about pain before touching the patient.
R Right-sided approach to the patient, whenever possible.
S Start at the foot of the bed; Similar structures on both sides of the body should be compared; Stethoscope diaphragm should be tapped to check it is not switched to the bell; Stethoscope and any other object that will touch the patient's skin (including hands) should be warmed and sterile; Say thank you on completing the exam.

Inspection

General (ABC)

A Appearance – JACCOLT
  J Jaundice
  A Anaemia
  C Cyanosis – peripheral and central

C Clubbing
O Oedema
L Lymphadenopathy
T Thyroid problem, i.e. goitre

Well groomed? Attire suitable for time, place and environment? Skeletal abnormalities such as kyphosis, scoliosis, lordosis?

B Behaviour – Comfortable at rest? Involuntary or abnormal movements such as fasciculation, tics, tremors, writhing, limping?

C Connections – oxygen, nebuliser, non-invasive ventilation, ventilator, inhalers, cigarettes or nicotine supplements, sputum cup (check the contents), catheter bag, wheelchair, walking stick, Zimmer frame, roller frame, Medic-Alert bracelet, drug cardex, observation chart contains vital signs such as temperature, BP, pulse, respiratory rate, oxygen saturations, GCS, MEWS/PARS score

Speech
- Hoarse voice (laryngitis), pseudobulbar palsy (Donald Duck speech), dysarthria, dysphasia, dysphonia
  See Skin colour, p. 17

Dehydration (BODS)
B BP is less when they stand (postural hypotension).
O Orbits are sunken.
D Dry mucous membranes – a dry tongue can be due to mouth breathing.
S Skin turgor is decreased (pinched skin should return to normal in hydrated state) – in an adult male approximately 4–6 litres has to be lost before skin turgor is affected.

Nutritional status
- Body mass index (BMI), weight/height^2 measured in kg/m^2
  — Underweight <18
  — Normal 18–25
  — Overweight 26–29
  — Obese 30–39
  — Morbidly obese >40

Body odour
- Acetone/sweet breath (DKA)
- Activities – alcohol, tobacco, marijuana
- Halitosis
- Hepatic foetor (stale urine/ammonia)
- Malodourous (excess sweating, poor hygiene)
- Uraemic foetor (mice)

Facial appearance (spot diagnosis – this should direct your examination)

- Acromegalic
- Anorexic
- Chemosis (CO_2 retention)
- Down's syndrome
- Moon face (cushingoid), malar flush (mitral stenosis)
- Myotonic dystrophy (temporalis wasting)
- Scleroderma (pinched facial appearance)/butterfly rash (**SLE**)

Hair

- Hirsutism – excessive coarse hair in the female in a male pattern (face, trunk, limbs).
- Alopecia (hair loss) – alopecia areata can lead to total scalp baldness (alopecia totalis) or loss of all body hair (alopecia universalis).
- Hypertrichosis – excessive coarse hair not following the male pattern.

Lymph nodes

See Figures 1.2–1.4.

Thyroid gland

See Thyroid examination, p. 18

Breasts

See Breast examination, p. 12

Hands

It is useful to shake hands in order to establish a bond with the patient and also to elicit information such as temperature, sweatiness, tremors, Dupuytren's contracture, difficulty releasing grip:

- Anaemia, pallor of palmar crease.
- Bands – **Beau's bands**, multiple, unpigmented, transverse lines, from an illness severe enough to temporarily stop nail growth (shock, malnutrition, weight loss). **Mees' bands**, solitary, white, transverse

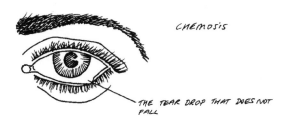

FIGURE 1.1

CERVICAL LYMPH NODES (CIRCULAR CHAIN)

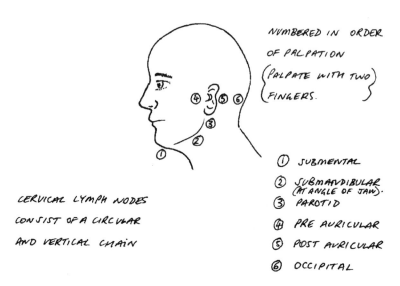

NUMBERED IN ORDER
OF PALPATION
(PALPATE WITH TWO
FINGERS.)

CERVICAL LYMPH NODES
CONSIST OF A CIRCULAR
AND VERTICAL CHAIN

① SUBMENTAL
② SUBMANDIBULAR (AT ANGLE OF JAW).
③ PAROTID
④ PRE AURICULAR
⑤ POST AURICULAR
⑥ OCCIPITAL

FIGURE 1.2

CERVICAL LYMPH NODES VERTICAL CHAIN

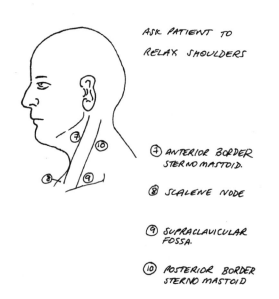

ASK PATIENT TO
RELAX SHOULDERS

⑦ ANTERIOR BORDER STERNO MASTOID.

⑧ SCALENE NODE

⑨ SUPRACLAVICULAR FOSSA.

⑩ POSTERIOR BORDER STERNO MASTOID

FIGURE 1.3

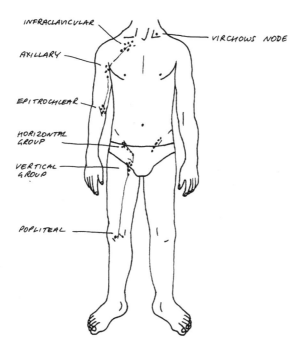

LYMPH NODES OF BODY

INFRACLAVICULAR
VIRCHOWS NODE
AXILLARY
EPITROCHLEAR
HORIZONTAL GROUP
VERTICAL GROUP
POPLITEAL

FIGURE 1.4

band (renal failure, chemotherapy, arsenic ingestion), **Muehrcke's bands**, multiple, opaque, transverse bands (hypoalbuminaemia, chemotherapy). *See* Nails, p. 15.

- Carpal tunnel syndrome
- Clubbing (*see* p. 14)
- Colour of nails (*see* p. 16)
- Dupuytren's contracture – fibrosis, contracture of palmar fascia (liver disease, epilepsy, trauma, elderly)
- Erythema of the palmar surface (cirrhosis, polycythaemia, pregnancy)
- Janeway's lesions – *see* Cardiovascular examination, p. 21.
- Koilonychia – spoon-shaped nails (iron deficiency, idiopathic – rarely)
- Onycholysis – distal nail separation (trauma, psoriasis, thyrotoxicosis)
- Osler's nodes – *see* cardiovascular examination, p. 21
- Pulse – character, rate, rhythm, left–right asymmetry between radial pulses, radiofemoral delay. *See* Pulse, p. 35.
- Pigmentation of palmar crease (Addison's, but normal in Asians, blacks)
- Splinter haemorrhages – small, linear haemorrhages under the nail. *See* Nails, p. 15.

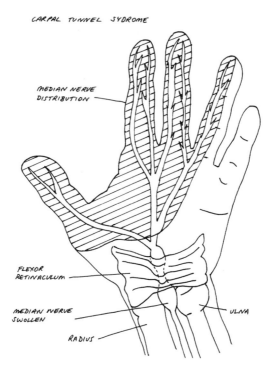

CARPAL TUNNEL SYDROME

MEDIAN NERVE DISTRIBUTION

FLEXOR RETINACULUM

MEDIAN NERVE SWOLLEN

RADIUS

ULNA

FIGURE 1.5

Abbreviated mental test

1 Time (nearest hour)?
2 Day of week?
3 Month?
4 Year?
5 Age?
6 Place?
7 Name three objects and advise that you will ask them to recall the objects after 2 minutes.
8 Date the Second World War started?
9 Name of the Prime Minister?
10 Count backwards from 20 to 1 (0 if any uncorrected mistakes).

Breast examination (NIPALLS)

This examination requires a lot of sensitivity. Male examiners may require a female chaperone. Cover the patient whenever possible.

N Nervous patient – try to place the patient at ease. Position the patient at 45 degrees.

I Inspect – look standing opposite the patient, ask them to sit with their arms relaxed at their sides.

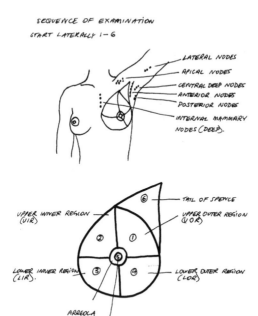

BREAST EXAMINATION

SEQUENCE OF EXAMINATION
START LATERALLY 1-6

LATERAL NODES
APICAL NODES
CENTRAL DEEP NODES
ANTERIOR NODES
POSTERIOR NODES
INTERNAL MAMMARY
NODES (DEEP).

UPPER INNER REGION (UIR)
UPPER OUTER REGION (UOR)
TAIL OF SPENCE
LOWER INNER REGION (LIR)
LOWER OUTER REGION (LOR)
ARREOLA
NIPPLE

FIGURE 1.6

P **P**alpate lump.
  — Ask the patient to point to the lump. Ask if it is tender. Start with the normal breast, palpating each quadrant with small circular flowing movements of the fingertips. This allows the breast to be rolled between the fingers and the chest wall. The lower quadrants should be bimanually palpated.
  — Palpate the problem breast, palpate the lump last. Feel for the following characteristics: site, size, shape, contour, consistency, tethering, temperature. Does the overlying skin move?
  — Ask them to raise their arms above their head.
  — Ask them to place both hands on their hips and push down. Now try to move the lump; if it is restricted then it is attached to muscle.
A **A**xilla – take the weight of the patient's arm to relax the axilla and examine from behind the patient. Palpate all walls of the axillae, medial, lateral, posterior, anterior, roof.
L **L**ymph nodes – palpate the cervical nodes and supraclavicular fossae.
L **L**iver and Lung bases.
  — Palpate the liver, is it large, knobbly, tender?

— Percuss the lung bases and auscultate for pleural effusions.
— Chest expansion, percussion, and vocal fremitus should be assessed.
S Spine – tap the spine gently to assess for metastatic infiltrations.

Inspection of the nipple (5Ds)
- Discharge
- Discolouration
- Dermatological changes:
  — Peau d'orange – orange-peel consistency? (tethering of skin)
  — Paget's disease of the nipple – eczema-like changes around the nipple, with discharge?
- Depression
- Deviation

Inspection of the breast
- Puckering? (skin drawn in)
- In-drawing of the nipple?
- Tethering of the nipple?
- Prominent veins?
- Look under large breasts for scars

Clubbing
Clubbing was first described by Hippocrates in 400 BC and is sometimes called Hippocratic fingers. The aetiology of clubbing is unknown; current research indicates it may be due to overproduction of PGE2, a compound that mediates the effects of inflammation. In normal individuals this is broken down by an enzyme 15-HPGD.
1 Staging of clubbing
2 Respiratory causes of clubbing (SLAM)
3 Cardiovascular causes of clubbing (CIA)
4 Gastrointestinal causes of clubbing (MICH)

Staging of clubbing (1–6)
- View fingernail from side – angle of base of nail is >160°
  1 Loss of normal 160° angle at base of nail – Schamroth's window test, or the diamond test: Ask the patient to hold the nails of their two index fingers together: if normal, will show a diamond-shaped window; if diamond is absent = Schamroth's sign.
  2 AP curvature increased
  3 Bouncy, spongy nail when examiner presses down on nail
  4 Drumstick-shaped fingertip
  5 Patient has wrist pain and wrist onion-skinning
  6 Hypertrophic pulmonary osteoarthropathy (HPOA)

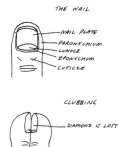

FIGURE 1.7

Respiratory causes of clubbing (SLAM)
S Suppurative lung disease (bronchiectasis, cystic fibrosis, empyema, lung abscess)
L Lung cancer
A Alveolitis (fibrosing)
M Mesothelioma

Cardiovascular causes of clubbing (CIA)
C Cyanotic heart disease
I Infective endocarditis
A Atrial myxoma

Gastrointestinal causes of clubbing (MICH)
M Malabsorption (coeliac disease)
I Inflammatory bowel disease (UC/Crohn's disease)
C Cancer, oesophagus, liver, bowel
H Hepatic cirrhosis

Nails
Bands
- **Beau's bands** – multiple, unpigmented, transverse lines, from an illness severe enough to temporarily stop nail growth (shock, malnutrition, weight loss)
- **Mees' bands** – solitary, white, transverse band (renal failure, chemotherapy, arsenic ingestion)
- **Muehrcke's bands** – multiple, opaque, transverse bands (hypoalbuminaemia, chemotherapy)
- **Splinter haemorrhages** – linear haemorrhages, run longitudinally along nails

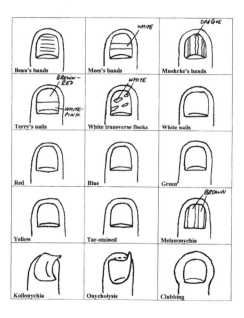

FIGURE 1.8

- Causes of splinter haemorrhages:
  — Anaemia (severe)
  — Haematological malignancy
  — Infective endocarditis
  — Sepsis (generalised)
  — Trauma
  — *Trichinella spiralis* infestation
  — Vasculitides (polyarteritis nodosa, rheumatoid arthritis, SLE).

Colours
- **Blue** – cyanosis, ochronosis, Wilson's disease (esp. lunulae of nails)
- **Blue-red** – polycythaemia
- **Green** – pseudomonas infection, fungal infection
- **Melanonychia** – multiple, brownish, longitudinal streaks (black patient – normal; white patient – melanoma under fingernails)
- **Red** – cherry red: CO poisoning)
- **Terry's nails** – distal half is brown-red, while proximal half is white-pink. (cirrhosis, chronic renal failure)
- **White nails** – leuconychia may be congenital or a sign of hypoalbuminaemia, which could be due to cirrhosis of the liver
- **White transverse flecks** due to minor trauma (striate leuconychia, this is *not* due to insufficient calcium)
- **Yellow** – nicotine stains, yellow-nail syndrome

Shapes
- **Koilonychia** – spoon-shaped nails (iron deficiency, idiopathic – rarely)
- **Onycholysis** – distal nail separation (trauma, psoriasis, thyrotoxicosis)

Skin colour
Physiological skin colouration is due to genetics and environment; there are many causes of pathological skin colour:
- Cyanotic, peripheral cyanosis (**COLD**), central cyanosis (**CLAMPS**)
- Hyperpigmented
- Abnormal melanin production
- Others

Cyanosis
Cyanosis occurs when there is >5 g/dL of deoxyhaemoglobin or <8 g/dL of Hb, or when oxygen saturation is less than 90%.

Cyanosis can be divided into peripheral (COLD) and central (CLAMPS).

Peripheral cyanosis, blue extremities (COLD)
C Central cyanosis always leads to peripheral cyanosis
O Obstruction of arterial supply (atheroma) or venous return
L Low cardiac output, heart failure, shock
D Damn cold! – vasoconstriction in fingers, Raynaud's phenomenon

Central cyanosis, blue lips (CLAMPS)
C Congenital heart disease (development of a right to left shunt)
L Lung pathology – massive PE, cor pulmonale
A Altitude (less oxygenated environment) or hypoventilation
M Metabolic (sulphaemoglobinaemia)
P Polycythaemia
S Shunt (right to left)

Hyperpigmented
- Addison's brown pigmentation
- Cushingoid (brown pigmentation in sun-exposed areas)
- Drugs – purple pigmentation following chlorpromazine
- Haemochromatosis 'bronze diabetes'

Abnormal melanin production
Underproduction
- **Patchy** (vitiligo) – melanocytes lost due to autoimmune illness
- **Total absence** (albinism) – genetic inability to form tyrosinase
- **Partial absence** (hypopituitarism) – pituitary has decreased ability to form melanin precursors

Overproduction
- **Melanocytic** – naevi, melanomas
- **Adrenal insufficiency** (Addison's disease) – pituitary produces increased amounts of melanin precursors
- **Pregnancy** – blotchy pigmentation of face (melasma/chloasma), increased pigmentation of the areolae, linea alba and genitalia due to oestrogen, progesterone and pituitary melanin precursors
- **Heavy metals** – iron overload (haemochromatosis)
- **Freckles, pigmented naevi** – local overproduction of melanin

Others
Human rainbow
- **Red** – erythema (superficial vascular lesions), port-wine stains
- **Orange** – hypercarotenaemia, excess dietary ingestion of β-carotene (from carrots)
- **Yellow** – jaundiced, yellow sclerae, mucous membranes and skin due to bilirubin retention, cholesterol deposition in xanthelasmas and xanthoma
- **Violet** – cutaneous haemorrhage, vasculitis; vascular tumours – Kaposi's sarcoma, haemangiomas; heliotrope eruption around eyes – dermatomyositis
- **Blue** – cyanosis
- **Pink** – carbon monoxide poisoning (due to excessive carboxy-Hb in the blood)
- **Plethoric** – polycythaemia/Cushing's syndrome (found in abdominal striae), plethoric facies in alcohol excess.
- **Pallid**, anaemia, shock
- **Uraemic** – grey/sallow
- **Black** – melanocytic (naevi/melanoma), black eschars (collection of dead skin)

Thyroid examination
Pre-examination checklist (WIPERS) Inspection
General
A **A**ppearance – nervous (hyperthyroid)
B **B**ehaviour – apathy, hypomania
C **C**onnections – glass of water

Hands and arms
- Carpal tunnel – fluid retention
- Thyroid acropachy – clubbing
- Plummer's nails – onycholysis – separation of nail from nail bed
- Pulse – hypothyroidism, slow with a low volume; hyperthyroidism, rapid, may be AF or arrhythmias
- Sweating (excessive) – hyperthyroid

- Tremor – accentuated by placing a piece of paper on the patient's outstretched hand
- Vitiligo (associated condition)

Face
- Eye signs – exophthalmos (sleeping with eyes open at night may lead to conjunctivitis, corneal abrasion and chemosis), exophthalmic ophthalmoplegia, lid retraction, lid lag
- Eyebrow – outer third is lost in hypothyroid
- Hair – greasy, lank in hyperthyroidism; coarse, dry and brittle in hypothyroidism

Neck
- Dilated veins over the upper part of the chest wall suggest retrosternal expansion of the goitre (thoracic inlet obstruction)
- Redness of the skin over the thyroid, suppurative thyroiditis
- Thyroid may be visible, goitre
- Thyroidectomy scar

Palpation
Before placing your hands on the patient ask if there is tenderness and be gentle. The neck is palpated from behind and then from the front. Palpate the thyroid gland with the patient's neck slightly flexed to relax the sterno-mastoid muscles. Place the fingers of both hands over the gland, feel for both lobes of the gland and its isthmus.

Estimate the size, and feel for the lower border of the thyroid; absence may signify retrosternal extension.

Features to consider
- Consistency – soft is normal; firm (simple goitre, Hashimoto's); stony hard (carcinoma, calcification, cyst, fibrosis, Hashimoto's); woody and tender (acute thyroiditis)
- Localised swellings may be better defined from the front
- Measure the size accurately in millimetres
- Mobility – carcinoma may tether the gland
- Shape – nodular or multinodular
- Tenderness – suggests thyroiditis

Palpation from front
Gently palpate any visible swelling to confirm visual impression of shape, size and surface.

Tracheal position
Check the position of the trachea (tip of two fingers in the suprasternal

notch). If there is extension of the thyroid mass below the suprasternal notch and the trachea is obscured then the thyroid cartilage must be examined. If there is a mass displacing the trachea it will tilt the thyroid cartilage laterally.

Palpate lymph nodes and drainage sites
- Primary drainage – deep cervical lymph nodes
- Secondary drainage – when primary overloaded – lymph nodes all over neck. Supra- and infraclavicular nodes, occipital, etc.

Percussion
Percuss the upper part of the manubrium to check for a retrosternal goitre, this is indicated by a change from resonant to dull.

Auscultation
Auscultate for bruits over each lobe of the thyroid (may occur in hyperthyroidism, and occasionally from the use of antithyroid drugs). Distinguish from carotid bruit (louder over the carotid), and venous hum (obliterated if a gentle pressure is applied over the base of neck).

Pemberton's sign
Ask the patient to lift both arms as high as possible. Is there a plethoric face, cyanosis or congestion. Respiratory distress and inspiratory stridor may occur. Distended neck veins indicate venous congestion. Test for thoracic inlet obstruction (due to a retrosternal goitre, lung carcinoma, other tumours – dermoid cysts, lymphomas, thymomas, or an aortic aneurysm) by auscultating for stridor whilst the patient takes in a deep breath.

Reflexes
Reflexes are very brisk in thyrotoxicosis and relaxation time is slower in hypothyroidism.

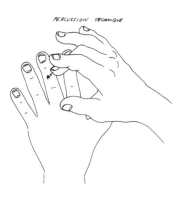

FIGURE 1.9

2

Cardiovascular system

Contents

- Examination: pre-inspection check, inspection (general, hands and arms, face, neck and JVP and chest)
- Chest: palpation
- Chest: auscultation
- Abdomen: palpation
- Feet
- Apex beat
- Heart sounds
- Murmurs
- JVP
- Pulse
- Congestive cardiac failure
- Infective endocarditis
- Marfan's syndrome
- Pericardial diseases
- Valve problems: aortic stenosis
- Valve problems: aortic regurgitation/incompetence
- Valve problems: mitral stenosis
- Valve problems: mitral regurgitation/incompetence

Examination

Pre-examination checklist (WIPERS) Inspection General

A **A**ppearance – cachexic, cyanotic, dyspnoeic, jaundiced, pallid (anaemia), hyperpigmented (haemochromatosis cardiomyopathy, addisonian hypotension) Syndromes: acromegaly (hypertension and cardiomegaly), ankylosing spondylitis (aortic regurgitation), Down's syndrome (PDA, ASD and VSD), Marfan's syndrome (aortic dissection, valve disease), Turner's syndrome (aortic coarctation, aortic stenosis).

B **B**ehaviour – comfortable at rest, leaning forward.

C Connections – oxygen, nebuliser, cigarettes or nicotine supplements, sputum cup (check the contents), cardiac monitor, ECG leads, drug cardex, observation chart contains vital signs such as temperature, BP, pulse, respiratory rate, oxygen saturations, GCS, MEWS/PARS score.

Hands and arms

- Anaemia – pallor of palmar creases.
- Aortic regurgitation – water-hammer pulse (the examiner places four fingers horizontally over the patient's palmar wrist, as they flex and extend their elbow).
- Arachnodactyly (Marfan's). *See* Marfan's syndrome, p. 40.
- BP
- Clubbing. *See* Clubbing, p. 14.
- Cyanosis. *See* Cyanosis, p. 17.
- Infective endocarditis lesions – Osler's nodes (0.5–1 cm red-brown painful subcutaneous papules on fingertips, palmar eminences).
- Janeway's lesions – painless palmar macules seen in IE. *See* Infective endocarditis, p. 38.
- Osler's nodes – red nodules approximately 5 mm in diameter, raised and tender. They are found on the pulps of toes and fingers and sometimes on the thenar or hypothenar eminences. Thought to be due to the deposition of immune complexes in IE. *See* Infective endocarditis, p. 38.
- Pulse – rate, rhythm, character, radiofemoral delay (coarctation of the aorta), radioradial inequality (atherosclerosis or thoracic artery aneurysm), radioapical delay (atrial fibrillation). *See* Pulse, p.x.
- Quincke's sign – the visible pulsation of red colouration seen in the fingernail bed in aortic regurgitation, blanching the nail makes this easier to see.
- Splinter haemorrhages
- Thyrotoxic – heat/tremor
- Xanthomata over extensor tendons (type II hyperlipidaemia) – pathognomonic of familial hypercholesterolaemia

Face

- Central cyanosis, blue mucous membranes
- Conjunctival pallor may indicate anaemia.
- Decayed teeth are a source of bacteraemia and potentially bacterial endocarditis.
- Exophthalmos, lid retraction (thyrotoxicosis)
- Eyes
- Corneal arcus – severe hypercholesterolaemia causes precipitation of cholesterol crystals at the periphery of the cornea
- Blue sclera – Marfan's, Ehlers–Danlos' syndrome (AR, ASD)
- Subluxated lenses – upwards: Marfan's; downwards: homocystinuria

- Argyll Robertson's pupil – syphilis
- Facies – apprehension, pain (angina, MI, PE, etc); cushingoid (HTN), acromegaly (CHF, HTN); Paget's (high output failure)
- High-arched palate – Marfan's syndrome. Investigate with a torch.
- Lid oedema – myxoedema, SVC syndrome, nephrotic syndrome, etc.
- Lips and sublingual – central cyanosis
- Malar flush, thin face, purple cheeks – mitral stenosis
- Ophthalmoscope – Roth's spots – small red haemorrhage with pale centre, due to vasculitis (IE)
- Xanthelasma – yellow periorbital plaques, can be a normal finding or may indicate type II or III hyperlipidaemia
- Yellow sclera – jaundice which could be due to hepatic engorgement due to cardiac failure, or haemolysis due to prosthetic heart valves especially mechanical valves

Neck and JVP and chest (J-SCAR)

Ask the patient to remove their top now or during chest exam. Cover woman's breasts with loose material.

J JVP (use R side) – inspect height, character, Kussmaul's sign (change on inspiration). The JVP gives an indication of the function of the right atrium and ventricle. *See* JVP, p. 30.

S Scars including sternotomy (midline) and mitral valvotomy (left lateral)

C Carotid pulse – inspect for carotid character and volume. Compress one carotid at a time. The carotid pulse gives an indication of the function of the aorta and the left ventricle.

A Auscultate the carotid pulse for a bruit, whilst the patient holds their breath.

R Respiration – using accessory muscles (pulmonary oedema, asthma, COPD)

Chest: palpation (PATS)

Ask the patient if any part is tender, examine that last.

P Pacemaker boxes

A Apex beat for presence, deviation, character. *See* Apex beat, p. 26.

T Thrills and heaves – a thrill is a palpable murmur. Place examining hand horizontally under the left pectoral, then vertically on the medial side of the left pectoral, then horizontally across centre of ribcage, below sternal notch. **Systolic thrill** coincides with apex beat. **Diastolic thrill** does not coincide with apex beat. **Parasternal heave** may be felt by placing the heel of the hand over the left parasternal region. If a heave is present it should lift the heel of the hand off the chest wall with each systole. Parasternal heaves are due to right ventricular hypertrophy or possibly severe left atrial enlargement pushing the right ventricle forwards.

S Sit the patient forward to examine the back. Is there Sacral oedema?

Deformities? Percuss for pleural effusions. Auscultate for effusions after auscultating the heart.

Chest: auscultation

Before auscultating remember that your dominant hand should hold the stethoscope whilst the other hand palpates the carotid pulse; if any murmur occurs in conjunction with a pulse it is systolic otherwise it is diastolic. The bell of the stethoscope is used to listen to low-pitched sounds (the murmur of MS); the diaphragm filters out these sounds and is used for high-pitched sounds (normal heart sounds and the murmur of AR).

Begin by positioning the patient at a 45-degree angle and auscultating the four valve areas with the diaphragm of the stethoscope in the following sequence: mitral area, tricuspid area, pulmonary area and then the aortic

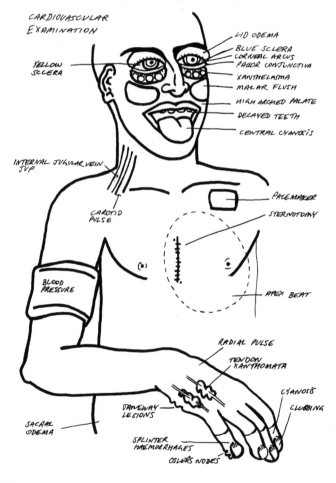

FIGURE 2.1

area. Also auscultate the carotids for bruits using the diaphragm, the patient momentarily holds their breath.

Ask the patient to roll onto their left side and relocate the apex beat and then auscultate the apex beat and axilla with the bell. Listen for the murmur of mitral stenosis.

Ask the patient to lean forward and hold their breath in exhalation, and with the bell of the stethoscope auscultate the tricuspid and aortic areas. Listen for the murmur of aortic regurgitation. (**RI**ght-sided murmurs are best heard on **I**nspiration and **LE**ft-sided murmurs are best heard on **E**xpiration.)

Auscultate the lung bases for bilateral basal crepitations, which may indicate heart failure. Unilateral basal crepitations indicate consolidation. Auscultate the abdominal aorta and renal arteries for bruits.

See Heart sound, p. 27.

Abdomen: palpation

- **Liver** – find, examine edge, pulsatile liver (tricuspid regurgitation), hepatomegaly (right heart failure)

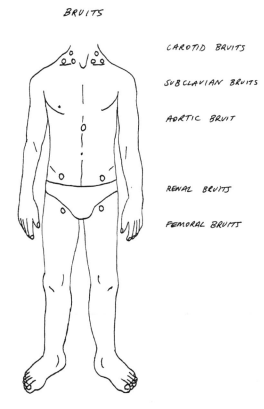

BRUITS

CAROTID BRUITS

SUBCLAVIAN BRUITS

AORTIC BRUIT

RENAL BRUITS

FEMORAL BRUITS

FIGURE 2.2

- **Spleen** – splenomegaly (endocarditis)
- **Abdominal aorta** – AAA

Feet (TOP)

T Tendon xanthomata on Achilles' tendon
O Oedema of ankles (right-sided heart failure)
P Pulses in feet – if not found move up sequentially to knees, femoral region
See Pulse, p. 35.

Apex beat

- Normal landmark
- Apex beat – differentials for impalpable apex beat (**DOPES**)
- Apex beat – abnormalities found on palpation (**HILT**)
- Apex deviation with trachea shift – mediastinal shift
- Apex deviation without trachea shift (**PICS**)
- Abnormal apex beat types (**D**ouble, **D**izzy, **D**ynamic, **K**inetic, **T**apping heart)

Normal landmark

- Find the sternal angle (angle of Louis) – level with 2nd intercostal space – count down to 5th intercostal space, 1 cm medial to midclavicular line

Apex beat: differentials for impalpable apex beat (DOPES)

D Death

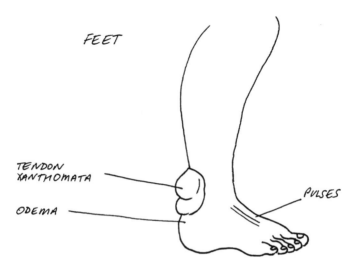

FIGURE 2.3

O Obesity
P Pericarditis/Pericardial tamponade/Pneumothorax
E Emphysema, other COPD
S Student incompetence/Scoliosis/Skeletal abnormalities (pectus excavatum)

Apex beat: abnormalities found on palpation (HILT)
H Heaving
I Impalpable
L Laterally displaced
T Thrusting/Tapping

Apex deviation with trachea shift
- Mediastinal shift

Apex deviation without trachea shift (PICS)
P Pectus excavatum
I Inversus, sinus
C Cardiomegaly
S Scoliosis

Abnormal apex beat types (Double, Dizzy, Dynamic, Kinetic, Tapping hearts)
- **Double** Double impulse – systole has 2 impulses (hypertrophic cardiomyopathy)
- **Dizzy** Dyskinetic – uncoordinated, easily palpable (MI)
- **Dynamic** Hyperdynamic – forceful, sustained apex beat (AS, HTN)
- **Kinetic** Hyperkinetic – coordinated, palpated beat is distributed over greater area (LV dilation)
- **Tapping** Tapping apex – S1 sound is palpable (mitral stenosis)

Heart sounds
1 Auscultation sites
2 Auscultation order
3 Heart sounds – S1, S2, splitting
4 Added sounds – S3, S4, opening snap, systolic click
5 Murmurs – general considerations, grading

Auscultation sites
(APTM) All Patients Take Medications or All People Take Marijuana

Anatomy of auscultation sites
- Aortic – 2nd right intercostal space
- Pulmonary – 2nd left intercostal space
- Tricuspid – 4th intercostal space, at lower left sternal border

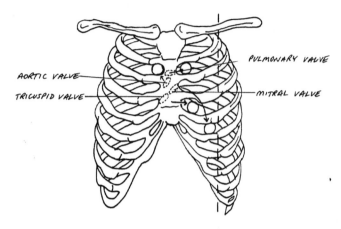

HEART AUSCULTATION SITES

PULMONARY VALVE

AORTIC VALVE

TRICUSPID VALVE

MITRAL VALVE

HEART VALVES ARE INDICATED WITH BROKEN LINES
AREAS OF AUSCULTATION ARE INDICATED WITH FILLED IN LINES

FIGURE 2.4

- **Mitral** – 5th left intercostal space, 1 cm medial to midclavicular line

Auscultation order
Always start at the apex (the mitral valve) and move upwards
- **Mitral** – bell and diaphragm
- **Tricuspid** – diaphragm
- **Pulmonary** – diaphragm
- **Aortic** – bell and diaphragm

Heart sounds
1st heart sound
- Mitral and tricuspid valves shutting
- **Louder** in MS, increased cardiac output, large stroke volume
- **Softer** in MR, decreased cardiac output, poor left ventricular function, long P-R interval (1st degree heart block)

2nd heart sound
- Has 2 parts – aortic valves shutting and then pulmonary valves shutting (A2, P2)
- **Loudness** of a component suggests it shuts with high pressure, indicating hypertension in the circuit. Aortic component loud = aortic HTN. Pulmonary component loud = pulmonary HTN.

- **Softer** in low cardiac output, calcification of aortic valve, AR.
- **Splitting of the 2nd heart sound** – either aortic valve shut early or pulmonary shut late:
    — Fixed splitting (unaffected by respiration) – ASD
    — Physiological splitting (increased normal splitting on inspiration)
    — Reverse splitting (widens on expiration) – AS, HOCM, LBBB, ventricular pacemaker.

3rd heart sound
Usually pathological after the age of 40. Early–mid diastole, low-pitched, 'gallop rhythm/triple rhythm' (heart failure + tachycardia + quiet first and second heart sound), louder on expiration.

Physiological
- Athletes
- Healthy young adults
- Pregnancy

Pathological
- Large poorly contracting left ventricle or MR

4th heart sound
Low pitch, best heard at the apex with bell of stethoscope, always pathological, caused by forceful atrial contraction therefore late diastole (presystole):
- Aortic sclerosis
- Block, heart
- Hypertension
- MI

Added sounds
Opening snap
A high-pitched click after S2 at apex – stiff mitral valve suddenly opened (MS).

Ejection systolic click
High-pitched click, soon after S1 followed by AS or PS murmur – stiff aortic valve suddenly opened (AS).

Midsystolic click
Mitral valve prolapse, may also have a late systolic murmur, best heard at the apex.

Mechanical heart valves
Opening and closing sounds, the former being quieter. High-pitched and maybe metallic sounding.

Pericardial rub
Indicates acute pericarditis, best heard at the left of the lower sternum with the patient exhaling. May be systolic and diastolic.

Pleuropericardial rub
It is of pleural origin and therefore affected by respiration.

Murmurs
- Murmurs – systolic and diastolic
- Murmurs – questions to answer on examination (SCRIPT)
- Murmurs – right versus left valves (RIPT and LEAM)
- Right versus left loudness (RILE)
- Murmurs – grading

Systolic or diastolic
- Systolic murmurs (**PASS**) – Pulmonary, Aortic Stenosis = Systolic
- Diastolic murmurs (**PAID**) – Pulmonary, Aortic Insufficiency = Diastolic
- Mitral and tricuspid murmurs are the opposite

Questions to answer on examination (SCRIPT)
S Site
C Character (harsh, soft, blowing)
R Radiation
I Intensity
P Pitch
T Timing

Right versus left valves (RIPT + LEAM)
- **RI** (Right) **P**ulmonary and **T**ricuspid valves
- **LE** (Left) **A**ortic and **M**itral valves

Right versus left loudness (RILE)
- **RI**ght-sided murmurs best heard on **I**nspiration
- **LE**ft-sided murmurs best heard on **E**xpiration

Murmurs: grading
Systolic murmurs are graded out of 6 and diastolic murmurs are rarely louder than a 4. The pathology of a murmur and the grading have no relation. Severe stenosis can have an inaudible murmur.

1 Only cardiologist can hear.
2 Trained doctor can hear in optimum conditions.
3 Easily heard. No thrill.
4 Loud murmur with a thrill.

5 Very loud. Thrill easily palpable.
6 Can hear murmur without a stethoscope.

Systolic and diastolic murmurs
Systolic murmurs
Systolic murmurs can be divided into ejection systolic and pansystolic murmurs.

Ejection systolic murmurs
- Can be due to increased stroke volume or normal/reduced flow through a stenotic valve

Causes of increased stroke volume:
- **ASD** (pulmonary flow murmur)
- **Athletes** (bradycardia therefore large stroke volume)
- **Fever**
- **Pregnancy** (cardiac output maximum at 15 weeks)

Causes of normal or reduced flow through stenotic valve:
- **Aortic stenosis**
  — Aortic sclerosis – can be differentiated from aortic stenosis because aortic sclerosis does not have the radiation to carotids, no change in BP, no slow-rising pulse, no ventricular hypertrophy.
- **Pulmonary stenosis**

Pansystolic murmurs
Are due to systolic leak from a higher- to a lower-pressure chamber.
- **Mitral regurgitation** – radiates to the axilla, is usually loud and blowing and is best heard at the apex.
- **Tricuspid regurgitation** – best heard at the left sternal edge and may be associated with a pulsatile liver and large v wave in the JVP.
- **VSD** – heard at the left sternal edge and associated with a thrill.

Diastolic murmurs
Diastolic murmurs can be divided into early-diastolic and mid-diastolic murmurs.

Early-diastolic murmurs
Aortic regurgitation – best heard at the left sternal edge (sometimes the right sternal edge if the aorta is dilated). Best heard with the patient leaning forward with the breath held in expiration. The murmur radiates to the back.

Pulmonary regurgitation – heard at the 3rd intercostal space on the left. Best heard with the breath held in expiration.

Mid-diastolic murmurs

Mitral stenosis – low-pitched and rumbling in character, best heard with the bell at the apex with the patient leaning to the left. The murmur begins after the opening snap.

Tricuspid stenosis – best heard at the lower left sternal edge and on inspiration.

Austin Flint's murmur – mid-diastolic murmur best heard at the apex – a low-pitched rumbling sound. Occurs in aortic regurgitation due to vibration of the anterior leaflet of the mitral valve as it is hit by blood jets from the left atrium and the aorta at the same time.

Graham Steell's murmur – best heard along the left sternal border on inspiration. It is due to pulmonary regurgitation in patients with pulmonary hypertension. It is high-pitched and has a decrescendo quality.

Carey Coombs' murmur – rare, only heard in rheumatic fever. It is soft and short and is due to vegetations on the mitral valve.

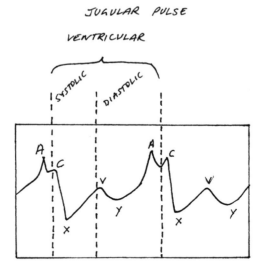

JUGULAR PULSE

VENTRICULAR

SYSTOLIC   DIASTOLIC

Ⓐ - ATRIAL SYSTOLE

Ⓒ - BEGINING OF VENTRICULAR SYSTOLE

Ⓥ - PEAK PRESSURE IN RIGHT ATRIUM AT OPENING OF TRICUSPID VALVE.

A - X = X DESCENT (FROM ATRIAL RELAXATION)

V - Y = Y DESCENT AT BEGINING OF VENTRICULAR FILLING

FIGURE 2.5

JVP

- JVP
- Function at waveform points (**ASK ME**)
- Distinguishing JVP from carotid (**FIND HA**)
- Examination of JVP
- Kussmaul's sign
- Hepatojugular reflux
- Causes of elevated JVP
- Causes of abnormal waveform

JVP

Acts as a manometer of right atrial pressure because there are no valves between the right atrium and the internal jugular vein. The external jugular vein is not examined because it is prone to kinking.

Function at waveform points (ASK ME)

A Atrial filling
S Systole
K Klosed tricuspid
M Maximal atrial filling
E Emptying of atrium

S1 occurs with 'a' and 'c' wave, S2 occurs with 'v' wave.

Distinguishing JVP from carotid (FIND HA)

F Fills from above
I Inspiration moves it (decreases in the healthy)
N Not palpable but visible
D Double pulsation for each arterial pulse
H Hepatojugular reflux
A Affected by posture (decreases as sit up more vertically)

Examination of JVP

Position at 45 degrees with head tilted upwards and laterally. Ensure good lighting.

Use the internal jugular, not external jugular. External jugular is lateral to SCM and easier to see. Internal jugular is medial/behind the clavicular head of SCM.

Normally JVP is not visible when sitting up. JVP >3 cm above sternal angle is pathologic. **JVP** has **3** letters.

Kussmaul's sign

Position the patient at 90 degrees. JVP increases on inspiration (constrictive pericarditis). Normal response is decrease of JVP on inspiration.

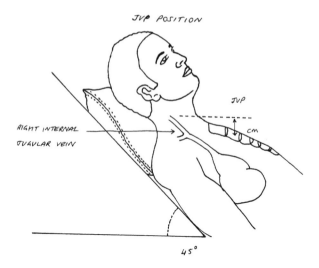

FIGURE 2.6

Hepatojugular reflux

This can be uncomfortable, only perform if strictly necessary.

Watch the JVP and press down on the liver for approximately 15 seconds. This causes an increase in venous return to the right atrium. In a normal person the JVP will rise transiently. However, if the JVP remains elevated it may indicate RVF.

Causes of elevated JVP (SHOT)

S Supraclavicular lymphatic enlargement
H Heart failure (right)
O Obstruction of vena cava – supraclavicular
T IntraThoracic pressure increase

Abnormal waveforms

- **Dominant a wave** (pulmonary stenosis, pulmonary hypertension, tricuspid stenosis)
- **Cannon a wave** (complete heart block, paroxysmal nodal tachycardia, ventricular tachycardia)
- **Dominant v wave** (tricuspid regurgitation)
- **Absent x descent** (atrial fibrillation)
- **Exaggerated x descent** (cardiac tamponade, constrictive pericarditis)
- **Sharp y descent** (constrictive pericarditis, tricuspid regurgitation)
- **Slow y descent** (right atrial myxoma)

Pulse
- Rate
- Rhythm
- Character
- Volume
- Delays
- Surface anatomy of pulses

Rate
Beats per minute: <60 = bradycardia; 60–100 = normal; >100 = tachycardia

Rhythm
Regular, regularly irregular, irregularly irregular (AF)

Character
- **Bounding pulse** – CO_2 poisoning
- **Collapsing pulse** (water-hammer pulse) – aortic regurgitation, heart block, PDA
- **Plateau pulse** – aortic stenosis
- **Pulsus alternans** (alternating strong, and weak beats) – LVF
- **Pulsus paradoxus** (volume decreases on inspiration by >10 mmHg) – constrictive pericarditis, tamponade, severe asthma
- **Small volume** – aortic stenosis, shock, pericardial effusion

Volume
Normal, high, low

Delayed pulses
Radioradial delay, radiofemoral delay – coarctation of aorta

Surface anatomy of pulses
- **Radial** – palmar surface of wrist, between flexor carpi radialis tendon and radius
- **Brachial** – cubital fossa, medial to biceps tendon
- **Carotid** – lateral to upper border of thyroid cartilage
- **Abdominal aorta** – in the midline, pressing at umbilicus. A large AAA may rupture if palpated without caution.
- **Femoral** – in the inguinal crease, below inguinal ligament, midway between ASIS and pubic symphysis (not pubic tubercle)
- **Popliteal** – best felt on flexing the knee, in the midline, on popliteal side of lower end of femur
- **Posterior tibial** – inferior to the medial malleolus, between flexor digitorum longus and flexor hallucis longus
- **Dorsalis pedis** – lateral to extensor hallucis longus, over tarsal bones

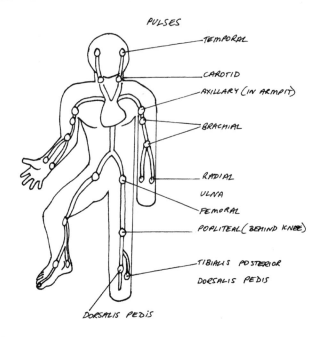

PULSES

TEMPORAL

CAROTID

AXILLARY (IN ARMPIT)

BRACHIAL

RADIAL

ULNA

FEMORAL

POPLITEAL (BEHIND KNEE)

TIBIALIS POSTERIOR

DORSALIS PEDIS

DORSALIS PEDIS

FIGURE 2.7

Congestive cardiac failure

Cardiac failure is where the cardiac output fails to meet the body's needs, despite normal venous pressures. The heart is a two-sided pump; when a side of the heart fails, there is a build-up of the column of blood behind it in the circuit. The pulmonary circulation is proximal to the left heart, and left heart failure (LHF) thus leads to pulmonary oedema. The systemic circulation is proximal to the right heart, and right heart failure (RHF) thus leads to peripheral oedema.

Right heart failure (RHF)

Causes of RHF
- Cor pulmonale
- LHF
- Tricuspid regurgitation

Symptoms of RHF
- Ascites
- Nausea
- Raised JVP
- Enlarged liver/spleen and kidneys
- Pitting oedema

RIGHT VENTRICULAR FAILURE

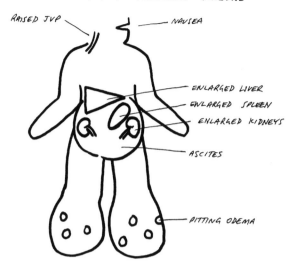

FIGURE 2.8

LEFT VENTRICULAR FAILURE

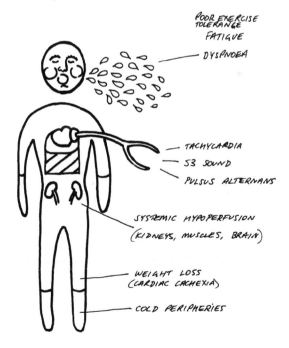

FIGURE 2.9

Left heart failure (LHF)

Causes of LHF

- Coronary artery disease
- Hypertension
- MI
- Mitral valve incompetence

Signs and symptoms of LHF

- Cold peripheries
- Dyspnoea
- Fatigue
- Poor exercise tolerance
- Pulmonary oedema (leads to) dyspnoea, paroxysmal nocturnal dyspnoea and cough productive of frothy sputum, sometimes pink
- Pulsus alternans
- S3 heart sound
- Systemic hypoperfusion, kidneys (poor urine output)/muscles (fatigue)/brain (confusion in elderly).
- Tachycardia.
- Weight loss (cardiac cachexia)
- Wheeze

Infective endocarditis

Well-known people with infective endocarditis

Composer Gustav Mahler, Scottish poet Robert Burns, physician Alois Alzheimer, actor Rudolf Valentino

Signs and symptoms of IE

- Anaemia
- Cardiac failure
- Cerebral infarcts
- Clubbing
- Dental work, braces
- Emboli (may cause abscesses in the affected organ, brain, heart, kidney, spleen)
- Fever, rigors, night sweats
- Immune-complex deposition, vasculitis can affect any vessel causing microscopic haematuria, glomerulonephritis, acute renal failure, Roth's spots (retinal haemorrhages with pale centres), splinter haemorrhages (on finger- or toenails, conjunctiva), Osler's nodes (painful infarcts on pulps of fingers and toes), Janeway's lesions (painless macules found on the palms, or soles of feet) are pathognomonic.
- Malaise
- Murmur, change in character or new

INFECTIVE ENDOCARDITIS

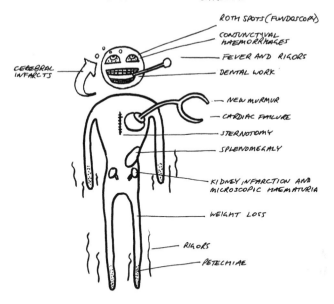

ROTH SPOTS (FUNDOSCOPY)

CONJUNCTIVAL HAEMORRHAGES

FEVER AND RIGORS

DENTAL WORK

CEREBRAL INFARCTS

NEW MURMUR

CARDIAC FAILURE

STERNOTOMY

SPLENOMEGALY

KIDNEY INFARCTION AND MICROSCOPIC HAEMATURIA

WEIGHT LOSS

RIGORS

PETECHIAE

FIGURE 2.10

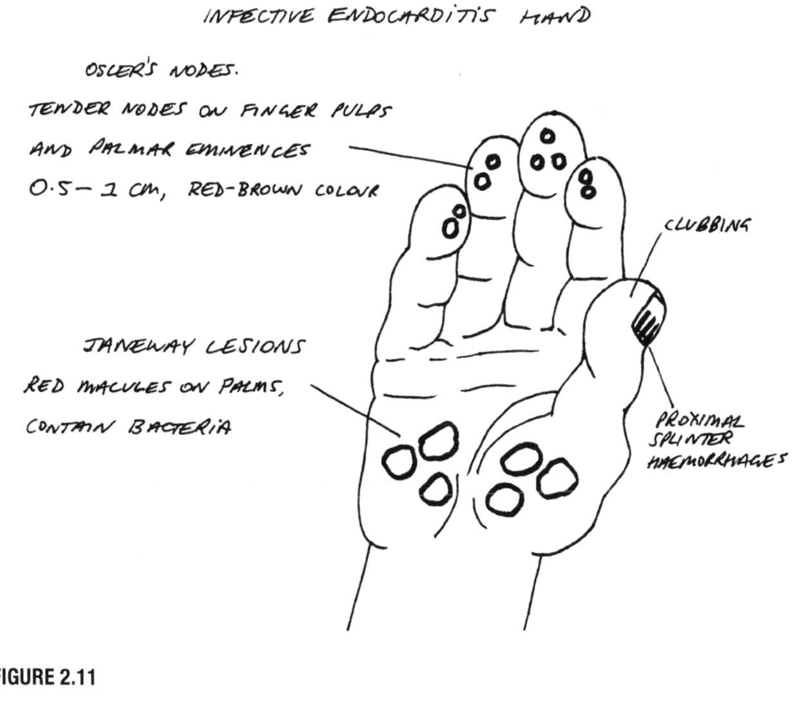

INFECTIVE ENDOCARDITIS HAND

OSLER'S NODES.
TENDER NODES ON FINGER PULPS
AND PALMAR EMINENCES
0.5 — 1 CM, RED-BROWN COLOUR

CLUBBING

JANEWAY LESIONS
RED MACULES ON PALMS,
CONTAIN BACTERIA

PROXIMAL SPLINTER HAEMORRHAGES

FIGURE 2.11

- Petechiae
- Regurgitant valve (any new murmur or change in an old murmur)
- Splenomegaly
- Valve disease
- Weight loss

Duke criteria for infective endocarditis
Definitive diagnosis is based on presence of:
- two major criteria, or
- one major and three minor criteria, or
- all five minor criteria.

Major criteria
- Blood culture positive for a typical organism in two separate cultures or persistently positive blood cultures, such as three >12 hrs apart
- Echocardiogram being positive (abscess, dehiscence of prosthetic valve or vegetation)
- Valvular regurgitation which is NEW (change in murmur is not sufficient)

Minor criteria (ETHIC)
- Echocardiogram that is positive but does not meet the major criteria
- Temperature being raised >38 degrees C
- History of predisposition (cardiac lesion, IV drug abuse)
- Immunological/vascular signs
- Culture (blood) that is positive but does not meet the major criteria

Marfan's syndrome
A connective tissue disorder with cardiological complications ranging from mild to severe. The diagnostic criteria of Marfan's syndrome were agreed in 1996 based on family history and a combination of major and minor indicators.

Well-known people with Marfan's syndrome
Composers Nicolò Paganini and Sergei Rachmaninoff, singer Joey Ramone, lead singer of the Ramones

Signs and symptoms of Marfan's syndrome
There are over 30 clinical features. Salient features are included below.

Cardiovascular system
- Angina pectoris
- Aortic aneurysm, dilated aorta, aortic dissection
- Cold peripheries from poor circulation

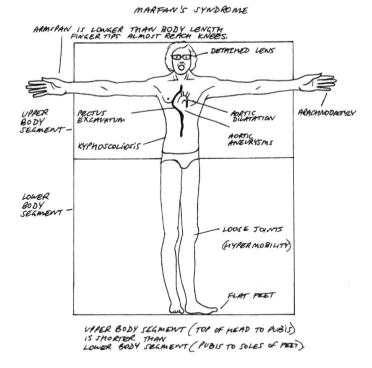

MARFAN'S SYNDROME

ARMSPAN IS LONGER THAN BODY LENGTH
FINGER TIPS ALMOST REACH KNEES.

DETACHED LENS

UPPER BODY SEGMENT—

PECTUS EXCAVATUM

KYPHOSCOLIOSIS

AORTIC DILATATION

AORTIC ANEURYSMS

ARACHNODACTYLY

LOWER BODY SEGMENT—

LOOSE JOINTS

(HYPERMOBILITY)

FLAT FEET

UPPER BODY SEGMENT (TOP OF HEAD TO PUBIS)
IS SHORTER THAN
LOWER BODY SEGMENT (PUBIS TO SOLES OF FEET).

FIGURE 2.12

- Regurgitation of aortic or mitral valves

Central nervous system
- Dural ectasia (weakening of the connective tissue of the dural sac) leading to lower-back pain, leg pain, abdominal pain, headaches

Eyes
- Detachment of the retina
- Near-sightedness (myopia)
- Astigmatism
- Subluxation of the lens

Pulmonary system
- Sleep apnoea
- Spontaneous pneumothorax

Skeletal system
- Above-average height
- Arachnodactyly (long fingers)

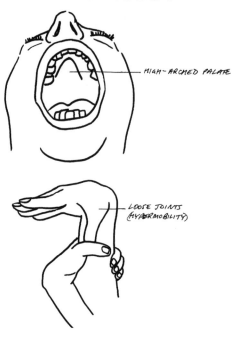

MARFAN'S SYNDROME '2

HIGH-ARCHED PALATE

LOOSE JOINTS
(HYPERMOBILITY)

FIGURE 2.13

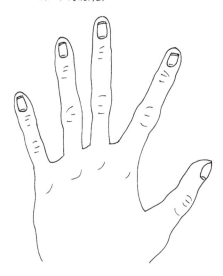

MARFAN'S SYNDROME '3
ARACHNODACTYLY

FIGURE 2.14

- Arm length is longer than height (dolichostenomelia)
- Crowded teeth
- Flat-feet
- Hammer-toes
- High-arched palate
- Joints are hyperflexible
- Pectus excavatum or pectus carinatum
- Scoliosis or kyphoscoliosis
- Thin wrists

Pericardial diseases
Well-known people with pericarditis
Singer Toni Braxton, singer Bob Dylan

Causes of pericarditis
- Dressler's syndrome
- Infection (viruses, bacteria, fungi)
- Malignancy
- Post MI (24–48 hrs)
- Radiotherapy
- Rheumatoid arthritis
- SLE
- TB
- Uraemia

Presentation of pericarditis (PERICarditis)
P Pulsus paradoxus
E ECG changes (saddle-shaped ST segment)
R Rub
I Increased JVP
C Chest pain (worse on inspiration, better when leaning forwards)

Beck's triad (cardiac tamponade) (3 Ds)
D Distant heart sounds
D Distended jugular veins
D Decreased arterial pressure

Valve problems: aortic stenosis (AS)
Causes of AS (REC)
R Rheumatic heart disease
E Elderly calcification of a tricuspid aortic valve (the most common)
C Congenital calcification of a bicuspid aortic valve

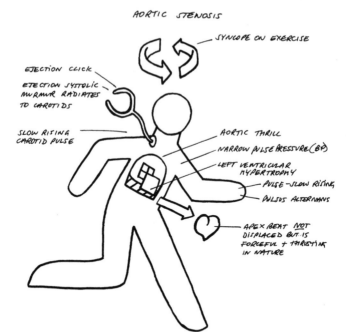

FIGURE 2.15

Presentation of AS (SADS)
S Syncope on exercise
A Angina
D Dyspnoea (exertional).
S Sudden death

Signs of AS
- Apex beat is not displaced, but is forceful and thrusting in nature (due to LVH), best felt with the patient sitting forward, on expiration
- Asymptomatic often
- Blood pressure (narrow pulse pressure)
- Ejection click may be heard from a bicuspid valve
- Ejection systolic murmur – heard loudest in the aortic area and radiates to the apex and the carotids
- Heart sounds – second heart sound is normally split in mild aortic stenosis, P2 preceding A2. As stenosis becomes more severe there is reversed splitting with A2 preceding P2. If there is calcification of the aortic valve then A2 will become softer and may be inaudible. Fourth heart sound (S4) may be present.
- Left ventricular outflow obstruction, left ventricular hypertrophy and enlarged coronary arteries

- Pulse is slow-rising, small volume, narrow pulse pressure – plateau pulse
- Pulsus alternans
- Slow-rising carotid pulse
- Thrill palpable in the aortic area
- **Aortic sclerosis** – can be differentiated from aortic stenosis because aortic sclerosis does not have the radiation to carotids, no change in BP, no slow-rising pulse, no ventricular hypertrophy.

Complications of AS (SLAMS)
S Sudden death
L Left ventricular failure
A Arrhythmias
M MI
S Stokes–Adams' attacks

Valve problems: aortic regurgitation/incompetence (AR)
Causes of AR
- Ankylosing spondylitis
- Aortic dissection
- Congenital
- Hypertension
- IE
- Marfan's syndrome
- Rheumatoid arthritis
- Rheumatic fever
- SLE

Signs of AR (acute presentation)
Acute left ventricular failure occurs when onset of aortic regurgitation is sudden (IE), because the left ventricle does not have time to adapt to the increased workload.
- Angina
- Austin Flint's murmur, low-pitched diastolic murmur
- Blood pressure (wide pulse pressure)
- Cyanosis
- Hypotension
- Palpitations
- Severe dyspnoea
- Tachycardia
- Weakness

Signs of AR (chronic presentation)
- Angina pectoris

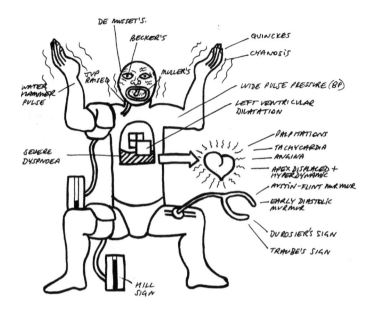

FIGURE 2.16

- Apex is **displaced and hyperdynamic** (left ventricular dilatation)
- Asymptomatic, often, due to adaptation of left ventricle to increased stroke volume
- Austin Flint's murmur
- Becker's sign – retinal arterioles show pulsation
- de Musset's sign – head-Duroziez's sign – systolic–diastolic murmur produced by compressing femoral artery with stethoscope
- Dyspnoea is a late feature and indicates left ventricle failure
- Early-diastolic murmur, high-pitched, best heard at 3rd and 4th intercostal spaces and also in aortic region at the apex
- Easily missed decrescendo diastolic murmur
- Ejection murmur, best heard in aortic area and radiates to carotid arteries
- Hill's sign – systolic pressure in the legs is raised in comparison to the arms by >100 mmHg (Hill's sign may be an artefact of sphygmomanometric lower limb pressure measurement).
- JVP is raised if there is heart failure
- Müller's sign – uvula has pulsation
- Quincke's sign – visible pulsation of red colouration in the fingernail bed. Blanching the nail bed makes this easier to detect
- Traube's sign – pistol shot auscultated over the femoral arteries in systole

- Water-hammer pulse (Corrigan's pulse) due to wide pulse pressure. Upstroke is abrupt and steep, peak is reached earlier than normal and there is a rapid downstroke. The amplitude is abnormally wide. With the patient lying back the examiner raises the patient's arm upwards and palpates the muscular part of the forearm and a tapping impulse is felt through the bulk of the muscles.

Valve problems: mitral stenosis (MS)

MS is a female title (**Ms**) and it is female dominant.

Causes of MS (CRAP)

C Congenital
R Rheumatic
A AND
P Prosthetic valve

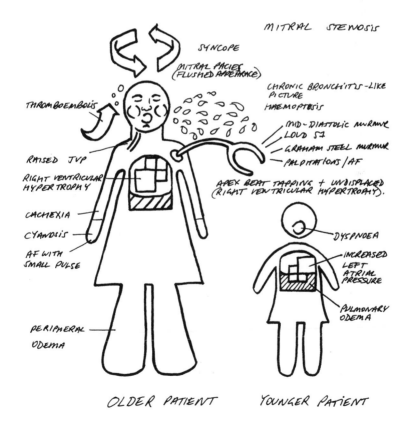

FIGURE 2.17

Presentation of MS

Can be of two types depending on the patient's pulmonary vascular resistance.

Normal pulmonary vascular resistance

Younger patients present with dyspnoea and pulmonary oedema due to increased left atrial pressure. This is exacerbated by situations of increased blood volume, such as during pregnancy.

Increased pulmonary vascular resistance

Older patients with low cardiac output and right heart failure present with fatigue, JVP is raised, mitral facies and right ventricular hypertrophy. Dyspnoea is less prominent in this group.

General presentation of mitral stenosis (MALAR PATCHES)

M Malar flush (cheeks)

A Atrial fibrillation is common, with a small pulse

L Left heart failure

A Apex beat is tapping, undisplaced (right ventricular hypertrophy)

R Right heart failure with a raised JVP

P Palpitations

A Auscultation – loud S1 with an opening snap and a rumbling mid-diastolic murmur heard best at the apex with patient on their left side and in expiration, Graham Steell's murmur is occasionally present

T Thromboembolism may be the first symptom

C Cachexia/Cyanosis/COPD or Chronic bronchitis-like picture (especially if left main bronchus is compressed causing bronchiectasis)

H Haemoptysis, rupture of congested bronchioles/Hoarse voice (massive enlargement of left atrium)

E Emboli (systemic) – risk of hemiplegia/patient in sinus rhythm is at risk of embolism

S Syncope

Valve problems: mitral regurgitation/incompetence (MR)

MR is a male title (**Mr**) and is more predominant in males.

Causes of MR

- Cardiomyopathy/congenital
- Ehlers–Danlos' syndrome
- Elderly calcification
- Functional (LV dilatation)
- IE
- Papillary muscle dysfunction/rupture
- Rheumatic fever/ruptured chordae tendineae

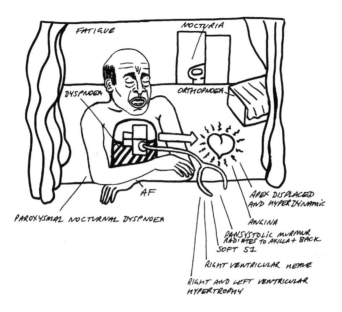

FIGURE 2.18

Signs of MR

- AF
- Angina on exertion – indicates ischaemic heart disease is likely to be the cause of the MR
- Apex is displaced and hyperdynamic
- Asymptomatic in mild cases
- Auscultation reveals soft S1 and splitting of S2 with a loud P2 (pulmonary hypertension) and a soft blowing pansystolic murmur with a reduced or absent S1 radiating to the axilla and back, best heard at the apex, especially in the left lateral position, with breath held in expiration
- Dyspnoea on exertion due to left ventricular failure
- Fatigue
- IE
- Orthopnoea
- Palpitations
- Paroxysmal nocturnal dyspnoea
- Right ventricular heave
- Ventricular hypertrophy, right and left.

3

Dermatology

Contents
- Dermatological history
- Dermatological examination
- Hallmark rashes and lesions
- Lesions nomenclature
- Elevated and non-elevated lesions
- Acne vulgaris
- Basal cell carcinoma (rodent ulcer)
- Cellulitis
- Herpes zoster
- Impetigo
- Lichen planus
- Malignant melanoma
- Molluscum contagiosum
- Necrotising fasciitis
- Psoriasis
- Seborrhoeic dermatitis
- *Staphylococcal* scalded skin syndrome
- Squamous cell carcinoma

Dermatological history
The history should include details of (**DOPES**):
D **D**uration
O **O**nset site, and spread from there
P **P**ersistence or fluctuation
E **E**xacerbating and alleviating factors
S **S**ymptoms such as blisters, burning, itching, odour, oozing, pain, soreness, weeping.

Other important features of the history include:

- **General health** at present
- **Past medical history**, particularly of atopy
- **Past history of skin problems**
- **Medications** used to try to treat the condition, together with any other medications taken and any allergies to drugs or contact allergens
- Family history – any skin disorders, in particular atopic disease or psoriasis
- Social history – including job, hobbies, travel and the interference of the condition with the quality of life

Dermatological examination
Pre-examination checklist (WIPERS) Inspection
General (ABC)

A Appearance – localised or generalised? Sites involved? Symmetrical or asymmetrical? Symmetrical rashes often suggest an endogenous process, psoriasis or atopic eczema. Asymmetrical rashes suggest exogenous aetiology, infection or contact dermatitis.

B Behaviour – comfortable at rest, painful, itchy

C Connections – antibiotics, anti-inflammatory medication, bandages, barrier cream

Inspect

S Shape and size
C Colour
A Arrangement
L Location
E Elevation and depression

Arrangement

- Arcuate – incomplete circle
- Annular – ring with dark edge, central clearing
- Digitate – finger-shaped
- Discoid – filled circle
- Discrete – areas separated by normal skin
- Disseminated – widespread discrete lesions
- Generalised – covers most of body, without intervening normal skin
- Grouped – multiple lesions grouped in one area
- Herpetic – blisters in groups
- Linear – arranged in a line
- Livedo – hatched pattern (vasculitis)
- Petaloid – merged discoids (seborrhoeic dermatitis)
- Polycyclic – merged circles (psoriasis)
- Reticulate – fine net-like pattern
- Serpiginous – snake-shaped
- Stellate – star-shaped (meningococcal septicaemia)

- Target – concentric rings (erythema multiforme)

Colour
- State colour
- Homogenous colour or graded

Elevation and depression
- Slope – edge from surrounding surface down to floor of ulcer – can slope inwards (venous ulcer), outwards (TB) or be vertical (non-healing)
- Ulcer – break in epithelial surface, extending to all layers of epithelium

Location (always describe in relation to anatomical landmark)
- Asymmetrical or symmetrical
- Exposed areas or covered
- Systemic rash
- Trunk or peripheral

Shape and size
- Note the shape and measure the size accurately in millimetres

Palpate the lesions
- Always ask the patient if they are tender before touching them
- Blanches with pressure, or not (purpura)
- Flat or raised
- Raised temperature indicates inflammation

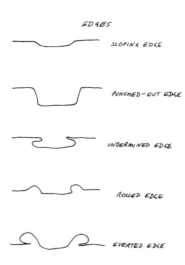

FIGURE 3.1

Texture of lesions
- Indurated – skin deeply thickened and hard – cutaneous metastatic cancer
- Lichenified – skin thickened with accentuation of normal skin markings from repeated rubbing
- Umbilicated – central indentation – usually viral, molluscum contagiosum, herpes
- Verrucous – irregular, rough surface – warts, seborrhoeic keratoses
- Xanthomata – yellow waxy lesions

Complete the examination
- Palpate nodes draining the lesions

Hallmark rashes and lesions
Location: facial
- Acne vulgaris
- Butterfly rash (SLE)
- DLE – sharp margins, on ears, lower lip, lower eyelid, nose
- Eczema
- Erythema infectiosum (fifth disease 'slapped cheeks')
- Measles – both appears and disappears from head to toe
- Rosacea – flushed, perhaps pustular
- Sarcoidosis – red-brown papules on eyelid, nostril rim

Location: palmar (PEGS)
P Palmar erythema (cirrhosis)
E Erythema multiforme – 'target lesions' (HSV, others).
G Gonococcus, meningococcus.
S Syphilitic lesions

Location: other (from scalp to feet)
- Ring around scalp – tinea capitis, aka ringworm – 'active' edge + central clearing + border of lesion shows scaling = ringworm
- Single dermatome – shingles
- 'Christmas tree' on back – pityriasis rosea
- Extensor side of elbows/knees, scalp, lumbosacral – psoriasis – Psilver Pscale over Psalmon Pskin = Psoriasis
- Flexor side of elbows knees – para-psoriasis, inherited eczema
- Between fingers – scabies
- Hands, feet, mouth – hand-foot-mouth
- Genitals and lips – herpes
- Groin, down upper thigh – tinea cruris
- Buttock and leg – Henoch–Schönlein's purpura
- Shins – erythema nodosum (infection of fat layer) – OCP, pregnancy, sarcoid, strep, drugs

- Legs/abdomen – erythema ab igne (heat rash)
- Foot – tinea pedis, (athlete's foot)

Lesion nomenclature
General lesions
- **Acanthosis** – thickening of the prickle cell layer of the skin
- **Acantholysis** – separation of epidermal cells due to dissolution of the intracellular cement substance
- **Atrophy** – skin is very thin and wrinkled – older people and those who use topical steroids
- **Blisters** – can be classified by size as:
  — Vesicles – less than 0.5 cm in diameter
  — Bullae – greater than 0.5 cm in diameter
- and according to the level of the histological split as:
  — Intra-epidermal blisters – thin-roofed and easily ruptured
  — Sub-epidermal blisters
- **Cicatrix (singular), Cicatrices (plural)** – a synonym of scar
- **Comedone** – plugged sebaceous follicle seen in acne vulgaris
- **Crust** – dried collection of blood, serum, pus – also called a scab
- **Erosion** – loss of epidermis
- **Erythroderma** – generalised redness of the skin affecting more than 90% of the body surface area – eczema, psoriasis, urticaria
- **Excoriation** – hollow crusted area caused by scratching
- **Granuloma** – discrete region of granulomatous inflammation defined by its histology after biopsy
- **Indurated** – abnormal hardening
- **Keloid** – scar that is very thick and raised
- **Lichenification** – rough thick epidermis with exaggerated skin markings
- **Macule** – <1 cm diameter, no elevation, non-palpable, may be erythematous or pigmented
- **Malar** – around zygomatic bones, aka cheekbones
- **Milia** – small (1–2 mm) whitish yellow papules frequently occur over the nose and face, may arise in areas of previously damaged skin, usually following blisters. May originate from maldeveloped sweat or sebaceous glands. Common and transient in the newborn. In later life they are more common in females and may be confused with xanthelasma around the eyes.
- **Moles** – localised collections of melanocytes. Those with potential for malignant change show altered pigmentation (increased or decreased), asymmetry, bleeding, enlargement, inflammation, irregularity of the surface or edge, itch, nodularity or ulceration.
- **Nodule** – elevated lesion >1 cm, rounded shape since thickness same as diameter
- **Papule** – <1 cm, palpable

- **Patch** – macule-like, but >1 cm
- **Papilloma** – a benign tumour caused by overgrowth of all elements of the skin. Comprising a core of connective tissue and blood vessels with a covering of skin epithelium. Usually less than 1 cm in diameter. May be pedunculated and smooth, soft, solid and of any shape. Frequently observed on the face and neck but may be found elsewhere.
- **Papillomatous** – warty, finger-like or round projections from surface
- **Patch** – a flat area of altered skin colour or texture, usually greater than 1 cm in size
- **Pedunculated** – on a stalk, having a narrower diameter at the base of the stalk
- **Plaque** – papule-like, but >1 cm
- **Pruritic** – itchy
- **Prurigo** – intensely itchy nodules that may be associated with an eczematous eruption. Individual prurigo nodule is a firm lump, 1–3 cm in diameter with a raised warty surface
- **Punctum** – central depression in papule – molluscum contagiosum
- **Scaly** – dry, horny build-up of dead skin cells, gross shedding of surface flakes
- **Scar** – discoloured fibrous tissue permanently replaces normal skin after destruction of dermis
- **Ulcer** – loss of epidermis and part of the dermis
- **Umbilicated** – elevated with central depression (molluscum contagiosum, HSV)
- **Whitehead** – keratin plug sealing off a pilosebaceous duct. The orifice of the pilosebaceous duct fails to dilate (in contrast to the formation of a **blackhead**) and the expanding plug ruptures the wall of the duct. This results in the release of the contents of the duct into the dermis where they excite an inflammatory reaction. This is seen in acne vulgaris.

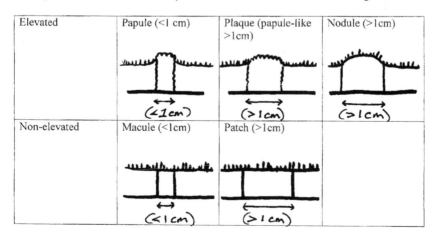

FIGURE 3.2

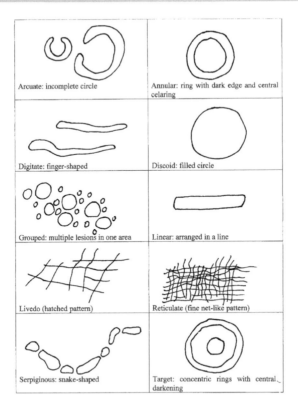

Arcuate: incomplete circle	Annular: ring with dark edge and central celaring
Digitate: finger-shaped	Discoid: filled circle
Grouped: multiple lesions in one area	Linear: arranged in a line
Livedo (hatched pattern)	Reticulate (fine net-like pattern)
Serpiginous: snake-shaped	Target: concentric rings with central darkening

FIGURE 3.3

Elevated and non-elevated lesions
Fluid lesions
- **Boil/furuncle** – tender, deep infection of skin
- **Bulla** – large vesicle
- **Carbuncle** – large furuncle
- **Cyst** – cavity lined with epithelium, and containing fluid, pus or keratin
- **Pustule** – pus-containing vesicle
- **Urticaria** – transient itchy swelling, due to dermal oedema (allergic response)
- **Vesicle** – fluid collection below epidermis
- **Weal** – small, elevated patch of dermal oedema, usually surrounded by a zone of erythema, <3 days

Blood lesions
- **Ecchymosis** – bruise – blue-black initially, from blood into tissue
- **Erythema** – flushing due to capillary dilation, redness that blanches on pressure (usually inflammatory)
- **Friable** – surface bleeds easily after minor trauma

- **Haemarthrosis** – bleeding into joints
- **Petechia** – pinpoint, dark-red, round, blood macule
- **Purpura** – a skin rash composed of petechiae, doesn't blanch on pressure
- **Telangiectasia** – localised dilated blood capillaries visible to naked eye, red, spidery, blanch on pressure

Pus-filled lesions
- **Abscess** – less than 1 cm in diameter, enclosed within a pyogenic membrane. Often caused by *staphylococcal* infection.

Acne vulgaris (ACNE V)
A Affects face, upper chest and back, especially in adolescents
C Comedone (blackhead) is main problem
N Normal skin commensal, *Propionibacterium acnes*, thrives in blocked follicles, inflammatory response to their presence causes the angry red appearance of inflamed lesions
E Excessive sebum production occurs under the control of androgens
V Variety of skin presentations, including comedones, red papules, pustules, nodules, cysts

Basal cell carcinoma (rodent ulcer) (RODENT)
R Rolled telangiectatic edge around the nodule
O Often found on the face
D Destructive locally if left untreated
E Excision is best for small lesions
N Nodule is pearly
T Tendency to occur in the fair-skinned

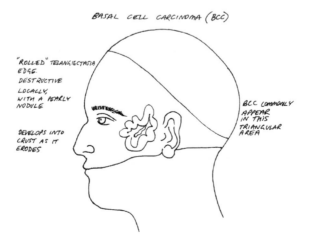

FIGURE 3.4

Cellulitis (SPREAD)

S Subcutaneous infection

P Portal of entry usually obvious (leg ulcer or wound)

R Red tender swelling

E Erysipelas presents very similarly and can be difficult to differentiate from cellulitis

A *Staphylococcus aureus* and group A streptococci usually cause the infection

D Defined edge of spreading erythematous oedema and vesiculation of erysipelas is absent

Herpes zoster infection, shingles (HERPES Z)

H Herpes zoster must be differentiated from Herpes simplex

E Eruption is polymorphic (red papules, vesicles, pustules and crusting)

R Recurrent infection is dermatomal in distribution, one or more dermatomes

P Primary infection is chickenpox

E Eruption may be preceded by symptoms of pain and malaise

S Scarring may occur with healing

Z varicella Zoster virus becomes dormant in the dorsal root ganglia

Impetigo (IMPETIGO)

I Infection with *Staphylococcus aureus*, *Streptococcus pyogenes* or both

M Mostly in young children

P Particularly around nose and surrounding parts of face

E Erythematous base with honey-coloured crusts

T Treat with Topical antibiotic such as fusidic acid for localised lesions

I Individuals are highly contagious from skin-to-skin contact

G Gram stain and culture of swab are diagnostic

O Oral flucloxacillin required for widespread impetigo

Lichen planus (PLANUS)

P Purple papules are flat topped and itchy

L Lacy markings on the surface of the eruption are known as Wickham's striae

A Aetiology is unknown, hepatitis C virus infection?

N Normally occurs at sites of trauma and affects flexor aspects of wrists, forearms, ankles and legs. Affects scalp (scarring alopecia), nails (longitudinal ridges), genitalia (annular lesions), mouth (on inner cheeks).

U Usually persists for 16–18 months

S Symptomatic treatment, topical steroids are used for severe itch

Malignant melanoma (MALIGNANT)

M Malignant melanomas develop from pre-existing moles in 30% of cases

A Adults with a new mole greater than 6 mm in diameter should seek advice

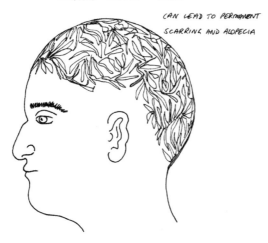

LICHEN PLANUS SCALP

CAN LEAD TO PERMANENT
SCARRING AND ALOPECIA

FIGURE 3.5

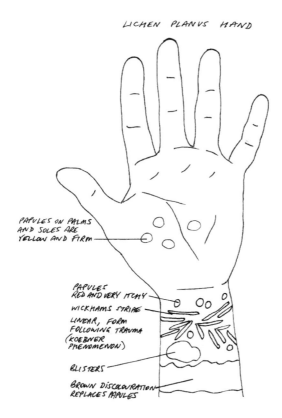

LICHEN PLANUS HAND

PAPULES ON PALMS
AND SOLES ARE
YELLOW AND FIRM

PAPULES
RED AND VERY ITCHY

WICKHAMS STRIAE

LINEAR, FORM
FOLLOWING TRAUMA
(KOEBNER
PHENOMENON)

BLISTERS

BROWN DISCOLOURATION
REPLACES PAPULES

FIGURE 3.6

L Local changes include inflammation, crusting, bleeding and sensory changes

I Irregular outline of mole from previously round or oval lesion is cause for concern

G Growing in size

N Non-uniform colour of mole with different shades of brown, black/red or blue is suggestive of malignant melanoma

A Altered size/shape/colour of pre-existing lesion suggests malignant melanoma

N Naevi/moles are the clinical differential diagnosis of malignant melanoma in young people

T Trunks of those older than 50 years frequently have seborrhoeic keratoses

Molluscum contagiosum, pox virus (POCS)

P Pink Papules with umbilicated central area

O Obtain a white cheesy material from the papule and microscope to confirm diagnosis

C Common in Children, Contagious and Caused by pox virus

S Spontaneously resolve

Necrotising fasciitis (FASCITIS)

F deep Fascia and vessels within it are affected

A group A streptococci are usually causative

S Secondary death of overlying skin

C Cellulitis-like appearance until 2 days into condition when lesion becomes purple, haemorrhagic bullae appear and tissue becomes necrotic

I Insufficient arteries and DM predispose to development but does occur in healthy individuals

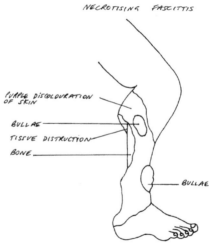

FIGURE 3.7

T Treatment is by urgent debridement and high-dose IV benzylpenicillin
I If untreated there is high mortality
S Skin loss is usually permanent

Psoriasis (PSORIASIS)

P Plaques are well defined
S Symmetrical plaques
O Onycholysis (distal separation from the nail bed) occurs in 2% of the UK population
R Red plaques
I Inflammatory skin condition, Immunologically mediated, TH1 cells predominate in early lesions
A Arthropathy develops in 7%
S Silvery Scale on plaques on extensor aspects of elbows, knees, Scalp and Sacrum
I In young patients very small plaques or guttate, pustular variants are seen on the palms and soles (Pustules, Sterile)
S Skin is treated with phototherapy (narrow-band UVB TL-01)

Seborrhoeic dermatitis (SEBORRH)

S Scaly eruption of unknown aetiology
E Eyebrows can be affected
B Based around face and head, on scalp causes dandruff, also found on nasolabial folds, cheeks and flexures
O Overgrowth of yeasts in skin could be a cause
R Responds to mild topical steroids and antifungal preparations
R Red in colour but can have a yellowish colour
H HIV-positive individuals can be affected quite severely

Staphylococcal scalded skin syndrome (SCALD)

S *Staphylococcal* toxins cause split in superficial epidermis
C Children especially infants are most susceptible
A A few days after initial infection there is sudden onset of widespread tender erythema and fever
L Layers of skin begin to detach in sheets
D Differential diagnosis is toxic epidermal necrolysis due to drugs

Squamous cell carcinoma (S CELL C)

S Sun-exposed areas are usually affected – ears, dorsum of the hands, bald scalp
C Crusted, firm, irregular lesion
E Excision used as treatment
L Lower lip can be affected in smokers
L Less likely to metastasise
C associated with Chronic inflammation such as venous leg ulcers

SEBORRHOEIC DERMATITIS

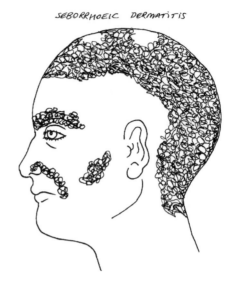

FIGURE 3.8

SQUAMOUS CELL CARCINOMA (SCC)

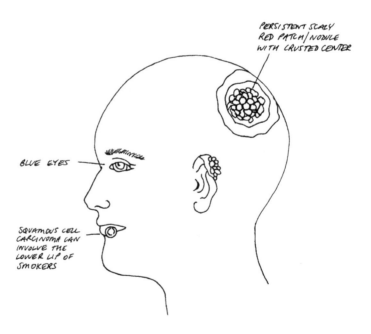

PERSISTENT SCALY
RED PATCH/NODULE
WITH CRUSTED CENTER

BLUE EYES

SQUAMOUS CELL
CARCINOMA CAN
INVOLVE THE
LOWER LIP OF
SMOKERS

FIGURE 3.9

4

Elderly care

Contents
- History
- Examination: inspection (general, hands and arms, face, eyes, mouth, ears, neck, back, heart, abdomen, feet, motor functions, percussion, auscultation)
- Mental state examination
- Alzheimer's disease

History (OLDER AND WISER)
Be mindful of the following mnemonic when taking a history from an older patient:

O 'Old dear' stereotyping is to be avoided – be respectful

L Lighting should be optimised to make your face more visible, avoid light glare

D Dentures, eyeglasses and hearing aids, if usually worn, should be used

E Extra time may be needed

R Reliability of the history may need to be determined with a Mental state examination (MSE), may require a collateral history

A Activities of daily living (ADLs), able to cope at home?

N Nutrition history including type, quantity, frequency[1]

D Depression, loneliness

W Weight loss (intentional or unintentional)

I Increased rate of urination, nocturia, dysuria[2]

S Social history/social supports/care givers

E Episodes of dizziness, falls

R Roids (haemorrhoids), indigestion, constipation, diarrhoea, melaena, PR bleeds

---

1 Patients having <2 meals a day are at risk of under-nutrition

2 UTIs are more common in the older age groups

Examination
Inspection
General (ABC)
A **A**ppearance – cyanotic, pallid (anaemia), hyperpigmented (haemochromatosis cardiomyopathy, addisonian hypotension), syndromes: Down's, Marfan's, Turner's

B **B**ehaviour – comfortable at rest, leaning forward

C **C**onnections – oxygen, nebuliser, cigarettes or nicotine supplements, sputum cup (check the contents), cardiac monitor, ECG leads, drug cardex, observation chart contains vital signs such as temperature, BP, pulse, respiratory rate, oxygen saturations, GCS, MEWS/PARS score, energy drinks/soft diet/NBM sign, walking stick/Zimmer frame/roller frame/wheel chair, glasses, catheter, hearing aid, IVI

Hand and arm
- Absent crescent-shaped lunula is a normal age-related finding
- AF
- Bruises (unexplained bruises could be due to abuse)
- Ecchymoses on forearm
- Liver spots
- Longitudinal ridges on nails are normal
- Refill of capillaries may show dehydration
- Steroidal skin

Face (HEAD)
H **H**airs (thin dermal) on ears, nose, upper lip and chin

E **E**yebrows drop below superior orbital rim

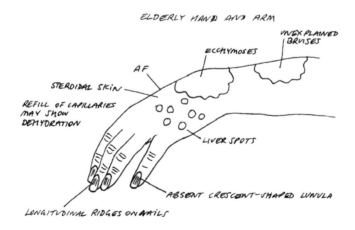

FIGURE 4.1

A **A**ge-related wrinkling of skin
D **D**ry skin

Eyes
- Acuity decreases
- Cataracts
- Entropion (in-turning of eyelid) ectropion (eversion of lower lid margins).
- Infection
- Light reflex decreases
- Presbyopia
- Senile arcus (arcus senilis) is a normal finding
- Small pupils (often an age-related change)

Mouth
- Angular cheilitis
- Cancer (leucoplakia, erythroplakia, ulcer, mass)
- Dentures should be removed to examine the mouth
- Erythema migrans (geographic tongue)
- Fissured tongue (xerostomia)
- Gums might bleed or be swollen

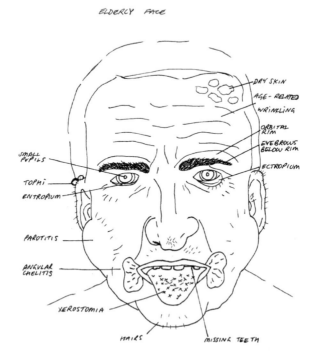

FIGURE 4.2

- Infections are usually fungal
- Parotitis (particularly in dehydrated patients, pus may be expressed from Stensen's duct when the interior of the mouth is palpated)

Ears (WAT?)
W Wax in the external auditory canal
A Aid (hearing) examined, battery might be dead if there is an absence of whistle (feedback)
T Tophi, normal age-related finding

Neck
- Check for full range of movement (ROM)

Back
- Osteoporotic fractures especially in the sacrum
- Scoliosis or kyphosis
- Tenderness of the spine could be due to metastatic infiltration

Heart
- Palpate the heart for cardiomegaly, lateral displacement of the apex

Abdomen
- Abdominal muscles weak? – may result in hernias
- Suprapubic tenderness, urinary retention secondary to prostatitis
- Should complete the examination with a PR

Feet (TOUCH IT)
- **T**rophic changes, venous eczema
- **O**edema (peripheral) due to heart failure
- **U**lcers, infected?
- **C**hronic cellulitis
- **H**allux valgus/hammer toe/claw toe
- **I**nfections, look between toes
- **T**hickened yellow toenail, onychomycosis (a fungal infection)

Motor functions (I Tickle Patients Get Really Cool Smiles)

I Inspection		
T Tickle	Tone	
P Patients	Power	Symmetrical is normal
G Get	Gait	Romberg's (+/-)
R Really	Reflexes	(+/-)
C Cool	Coordination	
S Smiles	Sensation	

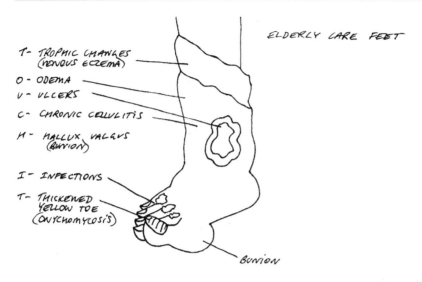

T- TROPHIC CHANGES (venous eczema)

O - ODEMA

V - ULCERS

C- CHRONIC CELLULITIS

H - HALLUX VALGUS (BUNION)

I - INFECTIONS

T- THICKENED YELLOW TOE (ONYCHOMYCOSIS)

ELDERLY CARE FEET

BUNION

FIGURE 4.3

Percussion
- Abdomen, lung bases

Auscultation
- Auscultate the heart for murmurs – systolic murmur is most commonly AV stenosis
- Auscultate the lung bases, any abdominal aneurysm, carotids and renal arteries

Mental state examination
- Orientation
- Registration
- Attention and calculation
- Recall
- Language

Maximum score is 30

Orientation
- Knowledge of time (1 mark each) – date/day/season/year/month
- Knowledge of location (1 mark each) – country/district/town/hospital/ward

Registration

- Ask patient to name three objects, such as pen, tie, cup (1 mark for each correctly identified object)

Attention and calculation

- Count backwards from 100 by 7s (1 mark each for first five correct)
- Not everyone has good numerical skills and therefore offer the option of spelling – spell DOCTOR backwards (1 mark for each correct letter).

Recall

- Patient is asked to recall the three objects they named in the registration section (1 mark for each correct item).

Language

- Patient is asked to follow a series of commands and is given 1 mark for each correct step: Take the paper in your right hand. Fold it in half. Put it on the table
- The patient reads the phrase 'CLOSE YOUR EYES' and can do it (1 mark).
- The patient reads the phrase 'WRITE A SENTENCE' and can do it (1 mark).
- Copy the design below – 1 mark is given if all angles present and figures intersect.

Alzheimer's disease (3As and 1E)

Well-known people with Alzheimer's disease

Actor Charles Bronson, artist Willem de Kooning, actress Rita Hayworth, actor Charlton Heston, author Iris Murdoch, former American president Ronald Reagan

Definition

An irreversible dementing illness due to the development of 'plaques' and 'tangles' in the brain. It is a clinical diagnosis and can only be definitively diagnosed as Alzheimer's on autopsy. Diagnostic criteria – amnesia and at least one of the following: (**3As and 1E**)

A Agnosia (cannot recognise people or objects although the senses are intact, **I-Knows-U?**)

A Aphasia (language problems – **A-Phrase-ia**)

A Apraxia (difficulty performing motor tasks, even though the physical ability to move the limbs and joints is normal – **Prax** is from the Greek word for Practical)

E Executive function (the ability to plan and organise)

5

Endocrinology

Contents

Endocrine history

Anxiety, appetite (increased or decreased), palpitations, polydipsia and polyuria, tiredness, tremor, weakness

Focal symptoms

Carpal tunnel syndrome (acromegaly, hypothyroidism, hyperparathyroidism), exophthalmos (if bilateral – Graves' disease), goitre, hair changes (hair thinning, hirsutism), headache, muscle or bone pain (fibromyalgia syndrome, polyarteritis nodosum, Takayasu's disease, Wegener's granulomatosis), pigmentation, skin changes, sweating (excess), visual field defects (or decreased acuity)

Hormonal changes

Altered libido (usually decreased), galactorrhoea, gynaecomastia, impotence, infertility, menses changes, puberty (delayed or precocious)

Examination
Pre-examination checklist (WIPERS)
Inspection
General

A **A**ppearance – stature (short, tall), sweaty (hyperthyroid, acromegaly, Addison's), weight (overweight – hypothyroid, Cushing's syndrome; underweight – hyperthyroid, DM)

B **B**ehaviour – comfortable at rest, anxious (hyperthyroid)

C **C**onnections – commode (diarrhoea – hyperthyroid, Addison's), drug cardex, observation chart contains vital signs such as temperature, BP, pulse, respiratory rate, oxygen saturations, GCS, MEWS/PARS score, energy drinks/soft diet

Perform a general examination keeping the following conditions in mind

- Acromegaly
- Addison's disease
- Cushing's disease
- Diabetes mellitus
- DKA
- Hypothyroidism
- Hyperthyroidism
- Graves' disease

Acromegaly
Definition
From the Greek *Akros* 'extremities' and *megalos* 'large'. Results from excess growth hormone production after epiphyseal plate closure at puberty.

Well-known people with acromegaly
Wrestler Andre the giant, actor Richard Kiel (Jaws in the James Bond films), actor Carel Struycken (Lurch in the Addams family)

Acromegaly history
Diabetes symptoms (polydipsia, polyphagia, polyuria – growth hormone is diabetogenic), enlarging hands, feet and facial features, fatigue, headache due to pituitary adenoma (commonly a superior bitemporal quadrantanopia, progressing to a bitemporal hemianopia) or due to skull enlargement and stretching of the dura mater, heat intolerance, impotence and reduced libido, sweating, weakness, weight gain, visual defects (pituitary adenoma), voice change.

Inspection and palpation
Hands and arms (OGRES POP)
O Oversized hands (compare with your own), spade hands with many wrinkles and skin folds

G Greasy (seborrhoea) and thick skin (gently pinch the skin of the dorsum of the hand)

R Rings feel tight

E Examination reveals carpal tunnel syndrome (soft tissue hypertrophy)

S Soft tissues of the palm may feel boggy and Sweaty

P Pulse (resting tachycardia – high output state)

O Osteoarthritis (premature)

P Proximal myopathy

Face (JAWS)
J Jaw is enlarged (prognathism), underbite

A Acne and greasy skin

W Widening of teeth (interdental separation)

S Supraorbital ridge is prominent (frontal bossing), Soft tissues are enlarged (ears, nose and lips)

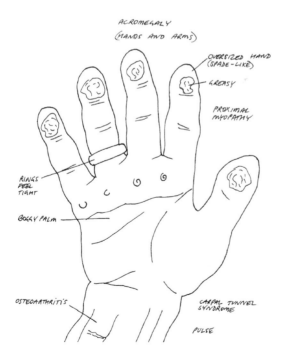

FIGURE 5.1

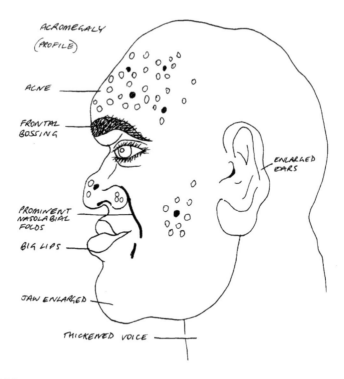

FIGURE 5.2

Eyes
Visual field defects (bitemporal superior quadrantanopia leads to bitemporal hemianopia)

Mouth (FILTH)
F Folds (nasolabial) are prominent
I Interdental separation of teeth
L Lips are big
T Tongue is enlarged (glossomegaly)
H Husky voice (thickened vocal chords)

Neck and axilla (GIANT)
G Goitre (multinodular)
I Increased JVP (congestive cardiac failure)
A Axillary acanthosis nigricans
N Neck soft tissue is enlarged
T Tags on skin (molluscum fibrosum) in the axilla

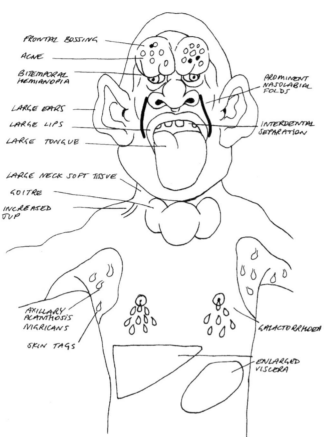

ACROMEGALY

FRONTAL BOSSING
ACNE
BITEMPORAL HEMIANOPIA
LARGE EARS
LARGE LIPS
LARGE TONGUE
LARGE NECK SOFT TISSUE
GOITRE
INCREASED JVP

PROMINENT NASOLABIAL FOLDS
INTERDENTAL SEPARATION

AXILLARY ACANTHOSIS NIGRICANS
SKIN TAGS
GALACTORRHOEA
ENLARGED VISCERA

FIGURE 5.3

Chest and abdomen (EGOES)

E Enlarged viscera (liver, spleen, heart)
G Galactorrhoea (spontaneous milk production)
O Oedema peripherally
E Enlarged feet
S Smell – increased sweating

Genitalia

N/A

Percussion

Lung bases for pulmonary oedema, enlarged viscera

Auscultation

Third heart sound (congestive heart failure), oedema (pulmonary – due to CHF)

Addison's disease
Definition
Addison's is due to inADequate cortisol. It can be chronic or acute (including the addisonian crisis).

Well-known people with Addison's disease
American president John F Kennedy, possibly Osama Bin-Laden, possibly author Charles Dickens

History
Chronic, non-specific vague symptoms
Anorexia, diarrhoea, loss of weight, mental changes, nausea, nocturia, seizures, skin pigmentation, tiredness

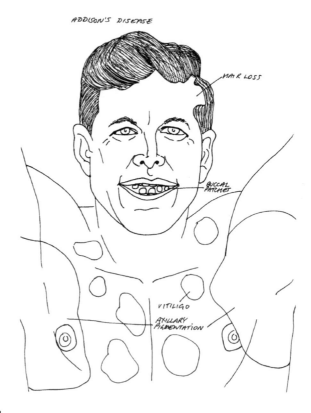

FIGURE 5.4

Chronic hypoadrenalism can be primary or secondary
- Primary – adrenal gland does not produce adequate amounts of adrenal steroid hormones
- Secondary – failure of ACTH production

Inspection
- Abdominal pain (intermittent)
- Amenorrhoea
- Anorexia (decreased appetite)
- Dehydrated
- Depressed affect
- Diarrhoea
- Diabetes mellitus (associated condition)
- Hypoglycaemia (reduced opposition to insulin action)
- Hypoparathyroidism (associated condition)
- Hypotension (postural), may cause dizziness and headache (due to ineffective catecholamine action)
- Hypothyroidism (associated condition)
- Impotence
- Lassitude
- Muscle weakness
- Nausea and vomiting
- Nipples show increased pigmentation
- Pigmentation, dull grey-brown colour, (only in primary hypoadrenalism due to melanocytes stimulated by increased ACTH levels), especially buccal, scars, skin creases, pressure points and nipples. If vitiligo is present this gives a patchy appearance.
- Premature ovarian failure (associated condition)
- Scalp, axilla and pubic regions have hair loss (androgen deficiency)
- Slow/lethargic/weakness
- Vitiligo (associated condition)
- Weight loss

Causes of acute hypoadrenalism
- Acute haemorrhagic destruction of both of the adrenal glands
- Adrenal crisis
- Drug related (inadequate dose)
- Iatrogenic – surgical removal of the adrenal glands
- Pituitary necrosis (Sheehan's syndrome).

Addisonian crisis (THE AD CRISIS)
T Tachycardia
H Hypotensive shock
E Eyes are sunken

A Abdominal pain/Anorexia/Anuria
D Dizziness especially postural/Dehydrated
C Cramps
R Rigid abdomen
I Increased calcium
S Serum Sodium is low
I Ill patient with a fever, who is vomiting
S Skin turgor is lost

Cushing's syndrome

Definition

Disorder due to excess cortisol in the blood (Cushing's is where cortisol is gushing). Cushing's disease is the most common form of Cushing's syndrome; it is due to increased pituitary ACTH secretion causing excess secretion of cortisol from hyperplastic adrenals.

History (STEROIDAL)

S Skin is steroidal and thin
T Thin arms due to Tissue wasting and associated muscle weakness (proximal myopathy – difficulty rising from squatting position) and pain (myalgia)
E Easy bruising and striae (red or purplish colouration)
R Reddened complexion (plethoric), elevated ACTH.
O Obesity *without* change in diet – trunk and abdomen, buffalo hump (supraclavicular fat pads) and moon face

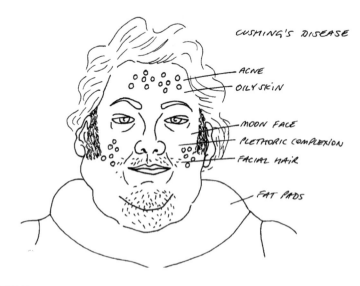

FIGURE 5.5

I Infertility, amenorrhoea (females), **I**mpotence (males)
D Diabetic symptoms; polyuria and polydipsia
A Androgenic symptoms – **A**cne, hair growth on body, frontal balding
L Lethargy which may be associated with depression, psychoses

Inspection and palpation
Avoid comparing the patient to a lemon or orange on matchsticks, in their presence.

Hands and arms (MATCHES)
M Myopathy (proximal) – ask them to put their arms in the air and say 'don't let me push your arms down' – gluconeogenesis leads to loss of muscle protein
A Arms are thin due to tissue wasting

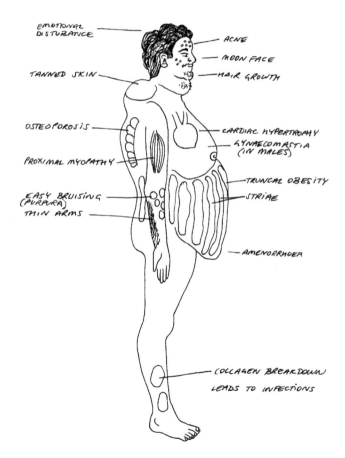

FIGURE 5.6

T Tanned skin in areas exposed to sunlight (in ACTH-dependent cases)

C Collagen breakdown in skin leads to poor wound healing with predisposition to infection

H Hair growth is excessive especially on the forearms

E Easy bruising (forearms and back of hands are common sites of minor trauma and may show purpura)

S Skin is steroidal and thin (gently roll the skin to assess skin-fold thickness, pinching may tear it)

Face and neck (MOONS)

M Mooning of the face (round face) – do not refer to it as moon face – it may cause offence

O Oily skin with acne (androgenic effects of steroids)

O Overgrowth of facial hair (androgenic effects of steroids)

N Neck and supraclavicular fossa have fat pads (it is not appropriate to refer to them as buffalo humps)

S Scarlet/plethoric complexion

Chest and abdomen (GO BEAST)

G Gynaecomastia in males

O Osteoporosis, pathological fractures, kyphosis

B Bruise easily (increased cortisol leads to collagen breakdown and thin skinning and fragile skin blood vessels)

E Excess hair

A Adrenalectomy scars

S Striae (purplish colour) also seen on breasts and thighs

T Trunkal obesity

Legs and feet

- oedema (salt and water retention due to excess cortisol)
- ulcers

Auscultation

- Wheezy or breathless (steroids may have been given for respiratory problem)

Diabetes mellitus (DM)

Definition

The body has a paucity of, or an insensitivity to, insulin resulting in cells being unable to absorb glucose and transform it into energy – therefore glucose accumulates in the blood leading to further pathology.

Well-known people with diabetes mellitus

Actress Halle Berry, musician Ella Fitzgerald, musician Elvis Presley, author HG Wells

Diabetes mellitus history (PPP)
P Polyuria (glycosuria causes osmotic diuresis)
P Polydipsia (dehydration leads to thirst)
P Polyphagia (fluctuating blood glucose levels)

Hypoglycaemia history
Morning headache, seizures, sweating, tremor, weight gain

Inspection and palpation
Head (ABCD)
A Acetone breath
B Blurred vision
C Cataracts and visual loss
D Deep breathing (Kussmaul's breathing)

Chest
Heart disease

Abdomen
Sites of insulin injection, lipodystrophy, necrobiosis lipoidica diabeticum, granuloma annulare, diabetic dermopathy, abdominal pain, weight loss, central obesity

Legs and feet
- Charcot's arthropathy
- Corns and calluses
- Decreased foot pulses

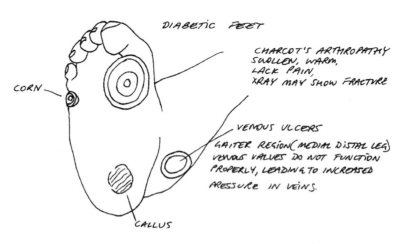

FIGURE 5.7

- Gangrene
- Peripheral neuropathy
- Ulcers, venous/arterial/mixed

Management: alphabet approach
A Advice (MR SHAHED)
B BP 130/85
C Cholesterol management <5
D DM, keep blood glucose between 4–7
E Eye checks
F Foot checks
G Guardian drugs (ACEi/aspirin)
H HbA$_{1C}$ <7%

Diabetic ketoacidosis (DKA)
A multisystem disease with microvascular and macrovascular complications.

Inspection and palpation (DKA)
D Dehydrated /drowsiness that can lead to coma
K Kussmaul's breathing/Ketoacidosis, K$^+$ (potassium) drops
A Acetone breath/Acidosis/Abdominal pain

Hypothyroid
Definition
Clinical syndrome due to deficiency of circulating thyroid hormones; in severe cases this leads to myxoedema where deposition of mucinous substances results in thickening of the skin and subcutaneous tissues.

Well-known people with hypothyroidism
Actress Kim Cattrall, presenter Kelly Osbourne, broadcaster Oprah Winfrey

Hypothyroidism history
Angina, anaemia (normocytic, normochromic), bradycardia, BP raised, cold intolerance, constipation, delayed puberty, depressed/mental slowness (cretinism in children), energy levels are low, lethargy, eyelids are swollen, impotence, infertility, malar flush, memory loss, menorrhagia, obesity, onset is insidious, psychiatric symptoms (myxoedema madness), skin and hair appear dry, hair loss on head, swallowing difficulties and hoarse voice due to goitre, tired.

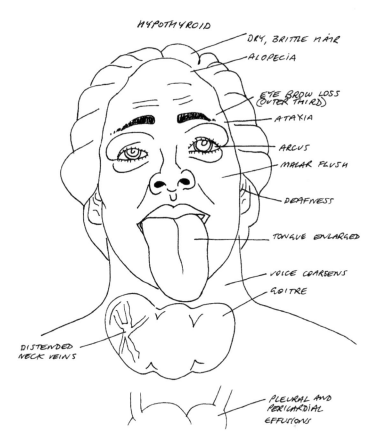

FIGURE 5.8

Inspection and palpation

Head

- Arcus (corneal)
- Cerebellar ataxia
- Deafness
- Dry, scaly and cold skin and dry, brittle, hair
- Eyebrows – loss of the outer third
- Goitre
- Inappropriate clothes (cold intolerance)
- Malar flush on a pale complexion
- Myalgia
- Obese
- Toad face (do not say this in front of the patient)
- Tongue is enlarged
- Voice, deepens, coarse

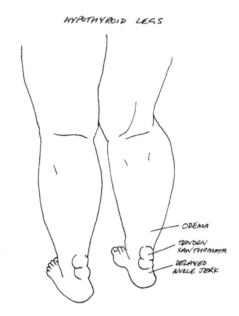

FIGURE 5.9

Hands and arms
- Bradycardia (examine pulse)
- Carpal tunnel syndrome
- Cold peripheries
- Examine pulse
- Oedema (non-pitting) especially eyelids and hands
- Tendon xanthomata

Neck and thyroid
Examine from the front and from the sides, inspect for:
- Distended neck veins
- Goitre (enlarged thyroid)
- Out (ask them to stick their tongue out)
- Scar (thyroidectomy)
- Swallowing, does the swelling move?

Palpation and auscultation
- Pericardial/pleural effusions/cardiac dilatation
- Abdominal ascites

Reflexes
- Delayed ankle jerk reflex

Hyperthyroid
Well-known people with hyperthyroidism
Former president of America George Bush, former first lady Barbara Bush

Thyrotoxicosis history
Activity is increased, amenorrhoea, appetite is increased, diarrhoea, emotional lability; irritability, exertional dyspnoea, goitre, described as swelling in neck, hair thinning, intolerance to heat, irritability, itch, muscle weakness, nervousness and palpitations, oligomenorrhoea, polyphagia, sex drive decreased, sweating, tremor, weakness, weight loss

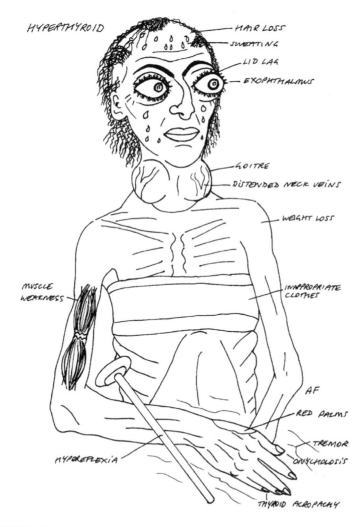

FIGURE 5.10

Inspection and palpation
Hand and arm (THYROID)

T Tremor

H Hot and sweaty

Y Y dressed like that? (thin clothes due to heat intolerance)

R Red palms (palmar erythema)

O Onycholysis (separation of the nail plate from the nail bed at its lateral and distal edges) – total separation is termed onychomadesis.

I Irregular pulse and tachycardia (fast AF)

D Drumstick fingers (thyroid acropachy) – this is clubbing with Graves' disease with extra swelling fingers and periosteal new bone formation.

Face, neck, thyroid, chest
- Examine from the front and from the sides, inspect for:
- Distended neck veins
- Exophthalmos (protruding eyes) –white sclera is exposed below the limbus
- Goitre
- Gynaecomastia in males
- Hair loss on the head
- Lid lag
- Lid retraction – being able to see the sclera above the upper limbus
- Out (ask them to stick their tongue out, does the swelling move)
- Swallowing, does the swelling move?
- Thyroidectomy scar?

Percussion
- Percuss the goitre for the lower limit of retrosternal extension

Auscultation
- Auscultate goitre for a bruit

Graves' disease
Definition
Autoimmune disease affecting the thyroid which can lead to its enlargement and overactivity

Well-known people with Grave's disease
Comedian Marty Feldman, poet Christina Georgina Rossetti

Inspection and palpation
Three signs unique to Graves' disease (TOP)

T Thyroid acropachy (clubbing)

O Ophthalmoplegia

P Pretibial myxoedema

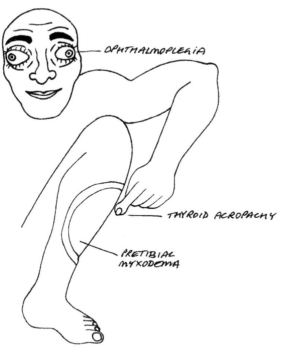

GRAVES DISEASE

OPHTHALMOPLEGIA

THYROID ACROPACHY

PRETIBIAL MYXODEMA

FIGURE 5.11

Thyroid eye disease (PROP)

P Proptosis (need to look from above, **PROP** on their shoulders to look down)

R Retraction (autonomic – may occur in any form of thyrotoxico)

O Ophthalmoplegia (upgaze palsy)

P Periorbital oedema and chemosis

6

Eyes

Contents

History
Presenting complaint
Onset – sudden or gradual, symptomatic or asymptomatic. Duration – transient or continuous, Location – unilateral or bilateral, focal or diffuse.

Eye history
Amblyopia, contact lenses, glasses, glaucoma, squint

Past medical history
Vascular conditions, (diabetes, hypertension)

Medications and allergies
Current medications including eye drops

Family history
Cataract, glaucoma, glasses, lazy eye, squint

Social history
Work in smoky or dark environment? Work in industrial environment with sparks or flying iron filings? Work in an office environment in front of computer for long periods of time?

Eye examination
Pre-examination checklist (WIPERS)
Inspection
General
A **A**ppearance – diagnostic facies (Marfan's, Down's)
B **B**ehaviour – pain (glaucoma)
C **C**onnections – reading glasses, dark glasses, white stick

Inspect both eyes and compare
- Asymmetry, deformities, discolouration, discharge, lesions, redness
- Brow – absent sweating (Horner's)
- Cornea – corneal arcus, Kayser–Fleischer's rings, lesion, scars, transparent or opaque
- Eyelids – blepharitis (pus on the eyelids), ectropion, entropion, xanthelasma
- Exophthalmos
- Iris – colour, defects
- Ptosis

Palpation
Ask the patient to look up and pull down both lower eyelids to inspect the conjunctiva and sclera.
- Conjunctiva – clear/infected – if conjunctivitis, wash hands immediately (adenoviral infection highly contagious)
- Sclera – injection, jaundice, pallor
- Spread each eye open with thumb and index finger. Ask the patient to look to each side and downward to expose entire bulbar surface. Palpate the eyeball for tenderness. Palpate the orbital rim for lumps.

Visual acuity
- Ask the patient to wear glasses or contacts if they usually wear them.
- Stand the patient 20 feet (6 m) from Snellen eye chart, or 14 inches (35 cm) away from a Rosenbaum pocket card.
- Ask the patient to cover an eye at a time and read as much of the chart as they can.
- Record smallest line read, e.g. 20/40 (6/12).

Visual fields
Visual fields can be examined with direct confrontation or more accurately with perimeters. The examiner keeps their head level with the patient's head and examines each eye separately. The patient and examiner cover eyes opposite to each other (right eye to left eye, etc.). Examine the outer aspects of the visual fields by wiggling your finger and ask the patient to say

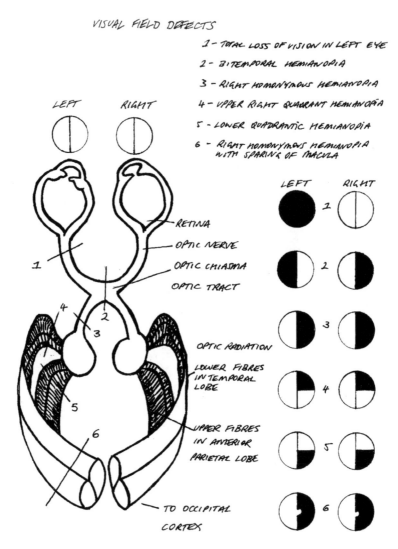

FIGURE 6.1

when they can see it moving (compare their perception with your own). Alternatively, map the visual fields using fingers.

The field for coloured targets is much smaller than that for white targets, and more sensitive to visual pathway pathology. Examine with a red hat pin and ask the patient to say when they can see the colour. Are there any scotomas?

Horizontal extent
160 degrees

Vertical extent
130 degrees

Physiological blind spot
15 degrees from fixation in the temporal field

Opthalmoscopy
Darken the room, adjust the scope so the light is no brighter than necessary.

Adjust aperture to a plain white circle. Set the dioptre dial to zero, or correct for your own vision. Assess the patient's right eye with your right eye and the patient's left eye with your left eye. Rest fingers on the patient's forehead and gently raise upper eyelid with thumb for stability.

Ask the patient to stare straight ahead at a spot on the ceiling or opposite wall. Look through the scope and approach the eye at a 45 degree angle. Firstly identify the retina which appears as a 'red reflex' – a dull/grey reflex indicates a cataract (or other opacity in the clear media). Adjust the dioptre dial as required to bring the retina into focus. Find a blood vessel and follow it to the optic disc.

Inspect optic disc
- Colour of disc – pale or pink?
- Margins – blurred or clearly defined?
- State of cup

Inspect vessels
- Inspect all four quadrants, veins appear darker than arteries
- Vessels engorged, attenuated, regular calibre, tortuosity

Inspect retina
- Haemorrhage, exudate, pigmentation, mass

Inspect macula
- Haemorrhage, exudate, oedema, drusen
- Foveal light reflex

Pupils
- **Shape** – relative size, irregularity
- **Light reaction** – assess both direct (same eye) and consensual (other eye) responses
- **Accommodation** – Ask the patient to concentrate on your finger which is held approximately 30 cm from their nose and then brought closer to their face. This can also be tested by asking the patient to alternate between looking into distance and then at a near target, e.g. hat pin or finger held 30 cm from the patient's nose.

Corneal reflections

Shine a light directly in front of the patient – corneal reflections should be centred over pupils.

Eye movements

Ask the patient to follow your finger with their eyes without moving their head. Test the six cardinal points in an H pattern.

Abnormalities of eye movements

- Failure of movement
- Fatiguability (myasthenia gravis)
- Gaze palsies (supranuclear lesions)
- Nystagmus

Corneal sensitivity (blink reflex)

Warn the patient that this can be uncomfortable; ask the patient to look into the distance. Touch the cornea with a wisp of cotton wool and check for a blink in both eyes. Repeat on the other side. Tests V sensory, VII motor.

Eye abnormalities

Common eye abnormalities

- Abnormal eye movements at rest
- Conjunctival injection
- Inequality of pupils (anisocoria)
- Orbital pulsation
- Ptosis (drooping of an eyelid)
- Widening/narrowing of the palpebral fissures

Pupillary abnormalities

Impaired pupillary reaction to light can be classified as afferent or efferent.

Afferent pupillary defect

- No direct light reflex
- Consensual reflex is present

Efferent pupillary defect

- Pupil is fixed and dilated with no reaction to light shone in either eye.
- Consensual reflex is present in the other pupil.

Parinaud's syndrome/pretectal syndrome

- Pupillary light response is lost but accommodation is preserved.
- Upgaze is lost.

Pupillary constriction (miosis)
Drugs
- Morphine and derivatives (parasympathomimetic)

Pontine haemorrhage causes bilateral pupil constriction
Horner's syndrome
- Unilateral miosis, ptosis, anhidrosis, enophthalmos (eyeball recedes into the orbit)

Pupillary dilatation (mydriasis)
Anxiety/excitement
- Causes bilateral dilated pupils.

3rd nerve/parasympathetic pathology
- Light reflex and accommodation are impaired due to a lesion in the ciliary ganglion.

Drugs
- Amphetamines and derivatives (sympathomimetic)
- Atropine (anticholinergic)

Pupillary reflexes
Direct light reflex
Constriction of the pupil on one side when that side is stimulated by light.

Consensual light reflex
Constriction of the pupil when the eye on the other side is stimulated by light.

Accommodation reflex
Viewing a nearby object (e.g. 10 cm) causes convergence of the eyes and bilateral pupillary constriction.

Ptosis
Ptosis is from the Greek meaning 'falling, fallen' and medically refers to droopiness of any body part. Ophthalmic term means drooping of the upper eyelid.

Causes of ptosis of the upper eyelid
- Aponeurotic ptosis – age-related, postoperative
- Congenital
- Myogenic ptosis – the muscles that raise the eyelid (levator palpebrae superioris and Müller's muscles) are not strong enough to do so. Myasthenia gravis, myotonic dystrophy, ocular myopathy

- Neurogenic ptosis – oculomotor nerve palsy (weak levator); Horner's syndrome (weak Müller's)
- Neurotoxic ptosis – bites by elapids such as cobras
- Pseudo-ptosis – empty socket or atrophic globe
- Upper lid tumours or oedema

Complications of ptosis
- Amblyopia
- Astigmatism
- Blindness

7

Gastroenterology

Contents

Gastroenterology examination
Pre-examination checklist (WIPERS)
Inspection

Expose the patient from nipples to knees, the parts not being actively examined can be temporarily covered with a cloth. Lay the patient flat, resting on a single pillow, with hands resting at the sides to relax the abdominal muscles. The examiner may need to kneel to perform the examination correctly.

General (ABC)

A **A**ppearance, anaemic (iron malabsorption, haemorrhage, ca.), jaundiced (liver disease), hyperpigmented (haemochromatosis), cachexic

B **B**ehaviour – comfortable at rest, anxious (alcohol withdrawal), mental state may be affected (hepatic encephalopathy, uraemic encephalopathy, hypoglycaemia, electrolyte disorders)

C **C**onnections, NG tube, drug cardex, observation chart contains vital signs such as temperature, BP, pulse, respiratory rate, oxygen saturations, GCS, MEWS/PARS score, energy drinks/soft diet, NBM

Hands

- Asterixis (PSE 2 degrees to alcoholism) – patient stretches out their hands and cocks them back with fingers spread out. Look for coarse flapping tremor (liver flap) involving wrist and MCP joints.
- Atheroma – palmar xanthomata, yellow deposits on palm of hand (type III hyperlipidaemia); tendon xanthomata, yellow deposits on dorsum of hand or arm, (type II hyperlipidaemia)
- Clubbing (UC or Crohn's, biliary cirrhosis, GI malabsorption). *See* Clubbing, p. 14.
- Dupuytren's contracture – contracture of palmar fascia, usually affecting ring finger (alcoholism, manual labour)
- Erythema of the palms (chronic liver disease, pregnancy, rheumatoid arthritis, thyrotoxicosis)
- Leuconychia (white nail), can be complete, streaks or spots. Can be congenital or acquired. Hypoalbuminaemia of chronic liver disease.
- Nails – koilonychia (iron deficiency 2° to GI bleeding), leuconychia (hypoalbuminism 2° to cirrhosis), Muehrcke's lines (hypoalbuminism 2 degrees to cirrhosis), blue lunulae (Wilson's). *See* Nails, p. 15.
- Pallor of palmar creases (anaemia 2 degrees to blood loss, malabsorption)
- Pyoderma gangrenosum on the dorsum of the hand (inflammatory bowel disease)
- Tar staining from smoking

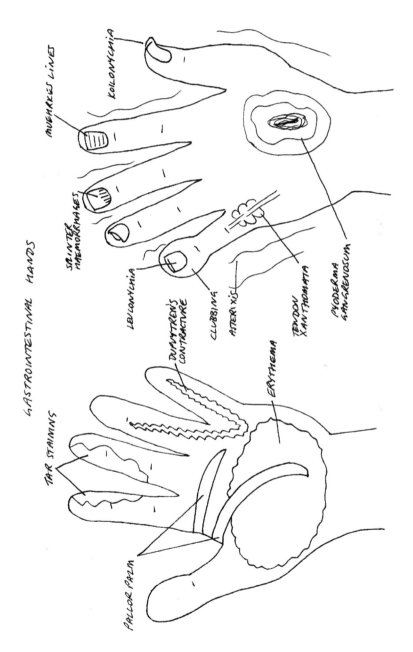

FIGURE 7.1

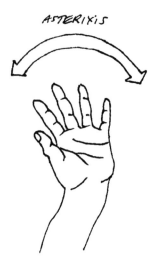

FIGURE 7.2

Arms (TIBS)

T Tuboeruptive xanthomata, yellow deposits on elbows, knees, (type III hyperlipidaemia)

I Itch, leading to scratch marks (deposition of irritating salts in the skin in jaundice)

B Bruising (decreased clotting factors 2 degrees to liver damage)

S Spider naevi (alcoholism)

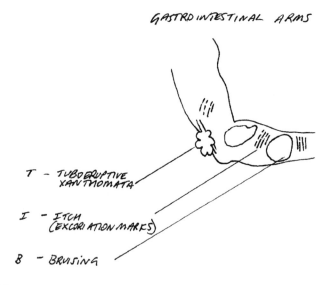

FIGURE 7.3

Face

- Anaemia
- Breath – foetor hepaticus (sweet faecal smell)
- Ethanol on the breath or foetor hepaticus (alcoholism)
- Eyes – jaundiced sclera, iritis (IBD), xanthelasma (yellow plaque periorbital deposits indicates elevated cholesterol), Kayser–Fleischer's rings (Wilson's disease)
- Lips – telangiectasis (Osler–Weber–Rendu)/brown freckles (Peutz–Jeghers')
- Jaundice – excess bilirubin
- Mouth – ulcers (Crohn's, coeliac disease)/white candida patches (can spread down the throat) cracks at the edges of the mouth (iron-deficiency anaemia), pigmented lesions – telangiectasias (Osler–Weber–Rendu), Peutz–Jeghers' spots
- Parotid enlargement (alcohol binges)
- Tongue – atrophic glossitis (smooth tongue) caused by B12 deficiencies, anaemia or sprue, black tongue (overgrowth of filiform papillae and accumulation of keratin), geographical tongue (may be normal or due to B12 deficiency), leucoplakia (Smoke, Spirits, Sepsis, Syphilis, Sore teeth)

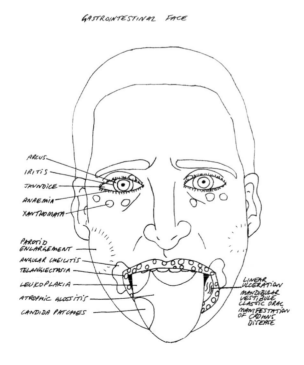

FIGURE 7.4

Neck, chest and back

- Acanthosis nigricans in the axilla, inguinal region, neck creases and below the breasts, (brown to black velvety papillomatous hyperplasia of the epidermis).
- Back – neurofibromas
- Enlarged cervical nodes – check the left supraclavicular node for Virchow's node (lung ca., GI malignancy), Troisier's sign (indicates stomach or less commonly lung malignancy).
- Gynaecomastia – chronic liver disease
- Secondary sexual hair loss

Abdomen

- Asymmetrical movement, ask the patient to take a deep breath in.
- Dilated veins – collateral veins can be secondary to IVC obstruction or in portal hypertension; they are usually tortuous dilated superficial epigastric veins. Cirrhosis of the liver can lead to caput medusa (dilated collateral veins radiating from the umbilicus). Flow direction – flows superior (IVC block), flows inferior (SVC block), navel radiation (portal hypertension)
- Enlarged abdomen – (Fat, Foetus, Faeces, Flatus, Fluid, Flipping-great tumour)
- Pulsations – AAA, peristalsis (seen in thin patients)
- Scars, stoma
- Shape and Symmetry of the abdomen – Sunken/Scaphoid abdomen
- Skin – Grey Turner's sign (acute pancreatitis) discolouration in flanks;
- Striae- regular striae (ascites, pregnancy, weight loss), purple, wide striae (Cushing's)
- Seborrhoeic warts, haemangiomas (Campbell de Morgan spots)
- Secondary sexual – hair, absence in adulthood indicates hypopituitarism, hypogonadism. Female distribution of body hair in the male could be secondary to cirrhosis. Male distribution of body hair in the female could be due to virilisation.
- Umbilicus:
  — Sister Mary Joseph's nodule (metastatic tumour)
  — Cullen's central discolouration (acute pancreatitis, extensive haemoperitoneum)
  — Everted umbilicus in abdominal distension

Palpation

Abdomen

Palpation can be divided into three parts, light, deep and palpation during respiration. Ask if the patient is tender anywhere and examine that part last. Kneel beside the patient so you are eye-level to the abdomen. Ask the patient to relax their abdomen (may require bending their knees) and place their hands palms up beside them. The patient will be more relaxed if they are warm and comfortable. Observe their face as you palpate the abdomen.

Light palpation

Gently palpate the abdomen by flexing your MCPs. Make continuous contact with the patient's abdominal wall to test muscle tone. Is there rigidity?

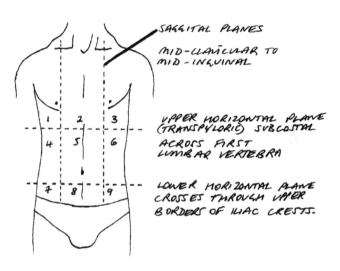

REGIONS OF THE ABDOMEN

SAGGITAL PLANES
MID-CLAVICULAR TO
MID-INGUINAL

UPPER HORIZONTAL PLANE
(TRANSPYLORIC) SUBCOSTAL
ACROSS FIRST
LUMBAR VERTEBRA

LOWER HORIZONTAL PLANE
CROSSES THROUGH UPPER
BORDERS OF ILIAC CRESTS.

THE ABDOMEN IS TRADITIONALLY DIVIDED INTO NINE REGIONS
BY THE INTERSECTION OF IMAGINARY PLANES, 2 HORIZONTAL
AND 2 SAGGITAL

    1 - RIGHT HYPOCHONDRIUM

    2 - EPIGASTRIUM

    3 - LEFT HYPOCHONDRIUM

    4 - RIGHT LOIN

    5 - UMBILICAL

    6 - LEFT LOIN

    7 - RIGHT ILIAC FOSSA

    8 - SUPRAPUBIC

    9 - LEFT ILIAC FOSSA

FIGURE 7.5

Test for rebound tenderness by pressing down into the abdomen firmly and then suddenly releasing the pressure. Rebound tenderness indicates deep-seated inflammation that has not caused guarding, the abrupt withdrawal has caused the sudden movement of the inflamed organ and thereby, pain. Generalised 'board-like' rigidity with little movement on respiration, and absent bowel sounds denotes peritonitis.

Deep palpation
Examine all nine quadrants systematically and feel for abnormalities in the underlying anatomy using the flat of the hand. Use the 'dipping technique' if there is pronounced ascites. The dipping technique causes the sudden displacement of liquid which in turns gives a tapping sensation over the surfaces of the liver and spleen, similar to the patellar tap.

Palpation during respiration
The following organs should be examined during inspiration, liver, gallbladder, spleen and kidneys.

Liver
Start at the RIF or at least at the transumbilical plane, ask the patient to breathe slowly. Keep your hand still during each inspiration, see if liver edge strikes radial edge of index finger. During each expiration, move your hand up by 2 cm.

Palpate liver surface, edge
- Smooth – normal, hepatitis, CCF
- Nodular – metastases, cirrhosis, tumour
- Pulsatile – tricuspid incompetence
- Tender – cardiac failure, hepatitis

Percuss the liver
Percuss down the right midclavicular line and find top border (normal – 5th rib in midclavicular line) and percuss downwards to find the lower border and then calculate the span. Normal span is 12.5 cm.

Gallbladder
Palpate the gallbladder by placing your fingers perpendicular to the right costal margin near midline. This is Murphy's point (costal margin in midclavicular line). Test for Murphy's sign – inspiration stopping upon palpation (acute cholecystitis).

Spleen
Palpate the spleen, begin at the right iliac fossa (RIF) and move diagonally towards the left upper quadrant (LUQ). Move up on inspiration and keep

your hand still when the patient breathes in. (The spleen and liver move downwards on inspiration due to the action of the diaphragm.) It might be necessary to roll the patient towards yourself to make the spleen more obvious. *See* Differentiating spleen from left kidney, p. 106.

Kidneys

This is sometimes incorrectly called balloting. Balloting only applies to a solid object suspended in a liquid medium. Place the heel of your left hand under the patient's right loin in the renal angle. Your right hand is placed on the patients RUQ. Flex your left MCPs in the renal angle so that your static right hand feels the impulse as the kidneys move forwards. Repeat for other side.

Pancreas

Palpate for a round, fixed, swelling above umbilicus that does not move with inspiration.

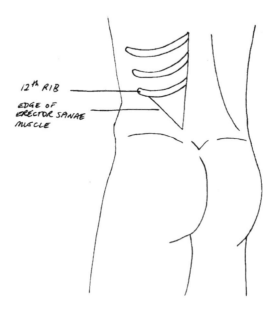

RENAL ANGLE

BETWEEN THE 12th RIB AND EDGE OF THE ERECTOR SPINAE MUSCLE

12th RIB

EDGE OF ERECTOR SPINAE MUSCLE

FIGURE 7.6

Aorta
Palpate in midline, superior to umbilicus. Place your two fingers on the outer margins of the aorta, fingers diverge (AAA).

Bladder
Ask the patient when they last urinated – the bladder is palpable if full, usually not palpable if empty.

Percussion
Abdomen
- Percuss the abdomen
- Bladder for enlarged bladder, pelvic mass
- Percuss masses

Ascites
Shifting dullness
Place your percussing finger vertically, so it points towards the patient's legs. Begin percussing at the midline and move medially towards yourself and mark the site of dullness with your finger or a non-permanent marker. Roll patient away from yourself so now lying on their left side, allow them to stay there for approx 30 seconds, then re-percuss while still lying on their left side. Ascites is identified if the dullness has moved (i.e. the point of dullness is now resonant, it has shifted).

Fluid thrill
Place your hands on each of the patient's flanks. Flick your hand on right flank, by quickly flexing MCPs and see if you can detect the resulting thrill on the left flank.

Auscultation
Bowel sounds
Bowel sounds – auscultate for 3 minutes (or until sounds are heard) below the umbilicus: *See* Bowel sounds, p. 105.

Abdominal aorta and renal artery bruits
- Arterial bruits are harsh systolic murmurs that arise from partially obstructed or narrowed arteries. Auscultate the abdominal aorta for a bruit (above the umbilicus).
- Auscultate the renal arteries for renal artery stenosis (right and left above the umbilicus).

Liver and spleen
Auscultate the liver and spleen for friction rubs – grating during breathing. In the liver it may indicate perihepatitis, Fitz-Hugh–Curtis' syndrome. A

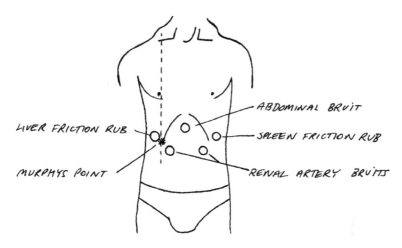

ABDOMINAL BRUITS

LIVER FRICTION RUB

MURPHYS POINT

ABDOMINAL BRUIT

SPLEEN FRICTION RUB

RENAL ARTERY BRUITS

FIGURE 7.7

splenic rub may indicate a splenic infarct or perisplenitis. The liver may have a bruit in liver cancer and alcoholic hepatitis. A systolic bruit may be heard over the liver in hepatoma.

Venous hum
Sometimes audible between the xiphisternum and umbilicus due to turbulent blood flow in a collateral blood supply that is well developed secondary to portal hypertension.

Succussion splash
Produced from a normal stomach up to two hours after food or drink. Otherwise it indicates delayed gastric emptying (pyloric stenosis).

Inspection
Legs (BOT)
B Bruising
O Oedema
T Tuboeruptive xanthomata, yellow deposits on elbows, knees (Type III hyperlipidaemia).

Complete examination
Examine the groin and lymph nodes, hernias and the external genitalia. Perform a PR examination; perform a PV in a female; dipstick the urine.

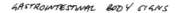

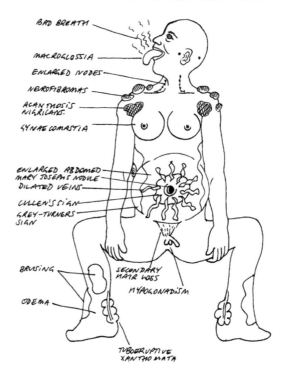

FIGURE 7.8

TRANSUDATE (PROTEIN <30 G /L)		EXUDATE (PROTEIN >30 G /L)	
HONC		**CAIB**	
H	Hepatic cirrhosis (portal HTN)	**C**	Carcinomatous infiltration of peritoneum
O	Ovarian tumour (Meigs' syndrome)	**A**	Acute pancreatitis
		I	Infection (TB, pneumococcal)
N	Nephrotic syndrome	**B**	Budd–Chiari's syndrome (inferior vena cava/hepatic vein obstruction)
C	Congestive cardiac failure		

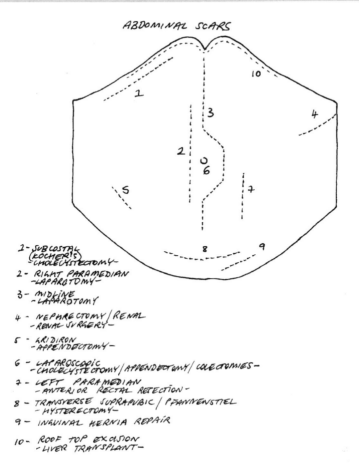

ABDOMINAL SCARS

1 – SUBCOSTAL
    (KOCHER'S)
    –CHOLECYSTECTOMY–
2 – RIGHT PARAMEDIAN
    –LAPAROTOMY–
3 – MIDLINE
    –LAPAROTOMY
4 – NEPHRECTOMY/RENAL
    –RENAL SURGERY–
5 – GRIDIRON
    –APPENDECTOMY–
6 – LAPAROSCOPIC
    –CHOLECYSTECTOMY/APPENDECTOMY/COLECTOMIES–
7 – LEFT PARAMEDIAN
    –ANTERIOR RECTAL RETECTION–
8 – TRANSVERSE SUPRAPUBIC/PFANNENSTIEL
    –HYSTERECTOMY–
9 – INGUINAL HERNIA REPAIR
10 – ROOF TOP EXCISION
    –LIVER TRANSPLANT–

FIGURE 7.9

Bowel sounds

- **Borborygmi** – normal bowel sound due to peristalsis
- **Ileus** – no bowel sounds for three minutes indicates bowel peristalsis has stopped. Ileus can be due to intra-abdominal inflammation/ infection or due to drugs (paralytic ileus)
- **High-pitched tinkling sound** – indicates obstructed bowel
- **Increased bowel sounds** (pronounced borborygmi) – small bowel obstruction, severe GI bleed, carcinoid syndrome

Differentiating palpable spleen from left kidney
Differences between the palpable spleen and left kidney (BEAN PISS)

		SPLEEN	*KIDNEY*
B	**B**ilateral?	No	Yes (in PKD)
E	**E**xtends beyond midline?	Sometimes	No (unless horseshoe kidney)
A	Can get **A**bove it?	No	Can get above it
N	**N**otch is present?	Yes	No notch is present
P	**P**ercussion note?	Dull	Not dull
I	**I**nspiration?	Moves superficially and diagonally	Moves vertically
S	**S**hape?	Smooth, regular	Polycystic kidneys are irregular
S	**S**ize?	Larger	Smaller size

Digital rectal examination (DRE)
- Introduction
- External inspection
- External inspection: straining
- Internal palpation

Introduction
'If you do not put your finger in you are putting your foot in it!' The PR examination is a vital component of an abdominal examination. Explain the procedure and ask permission. A male doctor should not perform a PR on a female patient unless he has a female chaperone. Ask the patient to lie in the left lateral position and draw their knees as close to their chest as they can. The examiner should wear gloves and place an encopad under the patient in case of mishaps. If the patient has an anal fissure a local anaesthetic suppository should be used before the PR is performed.

External inspection (FAT CRAPS)
F Fistula
A Anal fissure – be careful – this can be very painful
T Tags (normal, Crohn's, haemorrhoids)
C Carcinoma
R Rectal prolapse
A Anal warts
P Piles
S Signs of incontinence, diarrhoea

External inspection: straining

Ask the patient to bear down and observe for rectal prolapse upon straining, haemorrhoid? Prolapse? Incontinence? Ask if straining is painful.

Internal palpation

Lubricate your index finger and insert finger slowly, assessing external sphincter tone during insertion. In males palpate the prostate (anterior of rectum) it is normally smooth with a firm consistency and has a median groove between two lateral lobes. Assess size, shape, consistency and tenderness. Does it have a hard, irregular nodule (prostate cancer)? Is the prostate tender (prostatitis/prostatic abscess)? In females palpate cervix (anterior of rectum). Is there a mass in the pouch of Douglas?

Rotate finger, palpating all walls, ask the patient to bear down on your finger, feel the tone of the sphincter, can you feel a rectal prolapse? Can you feel haemorrhoids (not palpable unless thrombosed)? The rectum is smooth-walled, mucosal irregularity indicates carcinoma. An obstruction of the upper rectum may produce ballooning of the empty rectal cavity below. Withdraw finger and examine for stool (soft stool or hard impacted stool), pus, mucus, fresh blood, melaena – should be clean as a normal rectum is empty.

Enlarged kidney

Unilateral enlargement

- Compensatory hypertrophy due to renal agenesis, hypoplasia or atrophy affecting the other kidney
- Hydronephrosis
- Renal tumour

Bilateral enlargement

- Amyloidosis
- Horseshoe kidney
- Polycystic kidney disease

Inguinal canal

Indirect hernias	*Direct hernias*
80% of inguinal hernias	20% of inguinal hernias
Bilateral	Unilateral
Congenital	Acquired
Strangulate	Rarely strangulate
Pass through inguinal ring	Pass around the inguinal ring
Lateral to inferior epigastric vessels	Medial to inferior epigastric vessels
Outside Hesselbach's triangle	Inside Hesselbach's triangle

More common on right side, due to L1 damage during appendicectomy

Femoral hernias
- Inferolateral to pubic tubercle
- More likely to be irreducible than inguinal hernias
- **FEM**oral hernias more common in **FEM**ales

Hesselbach's triangle
- Inferiorly – inguinal ligament
- Laterally – inferior epigastric vessels
- Medially – rectus abdominus

Inguinal hernias
Anatomy (ICE)
I Internal spermatic fascia
C Cremasteric fascia
E External spermatic fascia

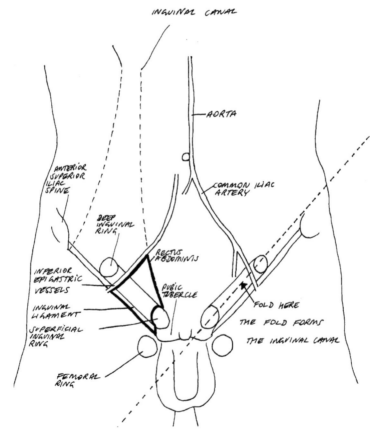

FIGURE 7.10

Differential diagnosis for inguinal hernias (MULLAHS)

M Muscle, (psoas abscess)
U Undescended or ectopic testis
L Lipoma
L Lymph nodes
A Aneurysm of femoral artery or saphena varix
H Hernia or hydrocoele
S Sebaceous cyst

Acquired (CANALS)

C Chronic cough/Constipation/COPD
A Ascites
N New and increased muscular effort; weight lifting
A Age has increased incidence
L Large size and body weight
S Sex – inguinal hernias more common in males and femoral hernias in females

Inguinal hernia examination (SCROTAL)

S Stand the patient up and observe from their Side, at eye level to the Swelling. Start with the normal side first. Support the patient's back.
C Cough please! Does a swelling appear? What is its relation to the pubic tubercle?
R Reduce the swelling (ask the patient to do this). 'You may need to lie down to do this Sir/Madam.'
O Once the patient is lying down and the swelling is reduced, Occlude the deep ring and ask the patient to cough. On releasing the pressure if a hernia appears it is an Indirect hernia. If a hernia appears whilst you are occluding the deep ring it is likely to be a Direct hernia.
T Transilluminate the swelling
A Auscultate the swelling, bowel sounds?
L Lymph nodes and testicles need to be examined, perform a PR to see if there is any obstruction that could be increasing intrathoracic pressure.
See Inguinal canal, p. 107.

Stools

Bristol stool chart

Type 1 – separate hard lumps, like nuts (hard to pass)
Type 2 – sausage-shaped, but lumpy
Type 3 – like a sausage but with cracks on its surface
Type 4 – like a sausage or snake, smooth and soft
Type 5 – soft blobs with clear cut edges (passed easily)
Type 6 – fluffy pieces with ragged edges, a mushy stool
Type 7 – entirely liquid

Bristol stool chart

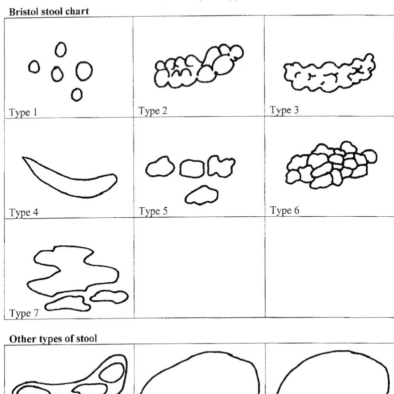

Other types of stool

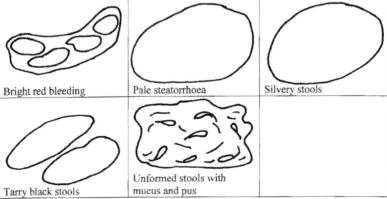

FIGURE 7.11

Types 1 and 2 indicate constipation
Types 3 and 4 are normal
Types 5–7 range from loose to diarrhoea

Bright red bleeding (from anal canal)
- Anal fissure (can be very painful during and after defaecation)
- Colorectal malignancy

- Colorectal polyps
- Diverticular disease
- Haemorrhoidal bleeding (can be profuse, may splash the toilet bowl and may continue after defaecation)
- Inflammatory bowel disease
- Ischaemic colitis

Excessive mucus production
- Colonic adenomas
- Colonic carcinoma

Pale (steatorrhoea)
- Fat malabsorption
- Pancreatic disease, small bowel disease

Silvery
- Steatorrhoea + GI haemorrhage (pancreatic carcinoma)

Tarry black (melaena)
- Upper GI bleed (peptic ulcers, caecal angiodysplasia) – can be difficult to flush away and foul smelling

Unformed stools with mucus and pus
- Colitis – may have urgency of defaecation

Urine colouration
- **Pale** haemolytic jaundice
- **Orange-brown** concentrated urine due to dehydration, conjugated bilirubin, rhubarb, senna
- **Red-brown** blood, haemoglobin, myoglobin, porphyrins, rifampicin, beetroot
- **Brown-black** bilirubin, melanin

Vomitus
Bilious vomiting
Yellow-green colour with bitter taste, regurgitation of duodenal content

Bright red blood in vomitus
Pharyngeal/oesophageal bleeding

Coffee-ground vomitus
Upper GI bleed, dark brown vomitus with silt-like sediment. These 'coffee-grounds' result from conversion of haemoglobin to acid haematin by gastric acid.

Dark red vomitus
May contain liver-like clots of blood are due to profuse bleeding, oesophageal varices, peptic ulcer.

Faeculent vomiting
Distal small bowel obstruction, colonic obstruction, gastrocolic fistula

Foul-smelling vomitus
Pyloric obstruction, stomach carcinoma, gastrocolic fistula

Projectile vomiting
Gastric outlet obstruction, leads to copious non bile-stained vomitus

Advanced chronic renal failure
- Arterial-venous fistula
- CAPD catheter
- Easy bruising
- Hypertension
- Lung crepitations
- Oedema
- Pallor
- Pericardial friction rub
- Peripheral neuropathy
- Peripheral oedema
- Pigmentation of nails
- Renal bruit if artery is stenosed
- Retinopathy
- Scratch marks
- Small kidneys found on ultrasound
- Yellow complexion (uraemic tinge)

Advanced liver disease
- Ascites
- Asterixis (flapping tremor)
- Cardiac disease
- Clubbing of fingers and maybe toes
- Dupuytren's contracture
- Easy bruising
- Foetor hepaticus
- Gastrointestinal haemorrhage
- Gynaecomastia
- Haemorrhoids
- Hepatomegaly and enlarged gallbladder
- Jaundice

- Leuconychia
- Lymph glands enlarged
- Mental state
- Needle marks (IVDU)
- Palmar erythema
- Peripheral oedema
- Salivary and parotid glands enlarged
- Scratch marks
- Spider naevi
- Splenomegaly
- Superficial abdominal veins
- Tattoos
- Testicular atrophy and sparse body hair

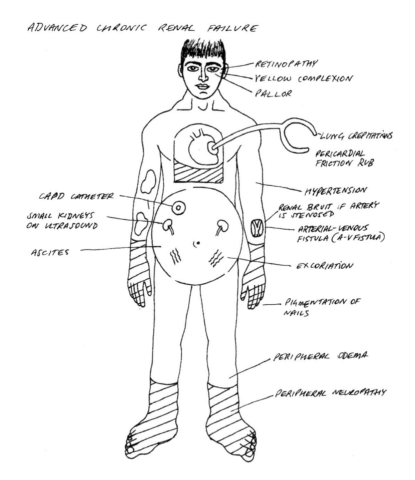

FIGURE 7.12

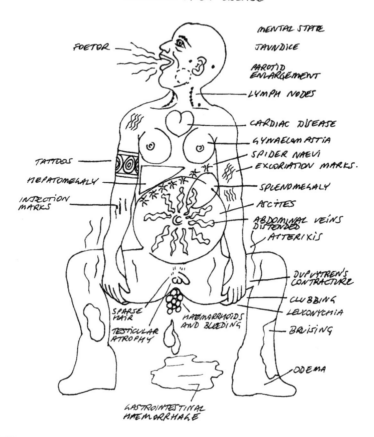

FIGURE 7.13

Haematuria

Painful

- Acute renal vascular disease
- Calculi (renal stones)
- Infection (UTI)
- Reflux nephropathy
- Renal papillary necrosis

Painless (GUSH)

G Glomerulonephritis
U UTI/Urogenital tumours
S Schistosomiasis/TB
H Hypertension

Haemochromatosis (iron overload)
Primary haemochromatosis
- Autosomal recessive
- Hyperabsorption of iron with parenchymal haemosiderin deposition in the adrenals, liver, pancreas, heart, testes, pituitary and kidneys
- Males of northern European descent
- Rarely recognised before the fifth decade of life

Secondary haemochromatosis
- Iron overload – can be due to chronic transfusion therapy for α-thalassaemia
- Alcoholics (alcohol increases iron absorption)

Haemochromatosis signs (Bronze-PATCH)
B Bronze skin pigmentation
P Pancreatic dysfunction
A Arthropathy of MCP joints
T Testicular atrophy
C Cardiac dysfunction (CHF)
H Hepatomegaly and abdominal tenderness

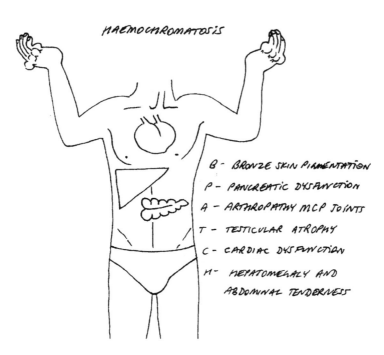

FIGURE 7.14

115

Hepatitis
Well-known people with hepatitis
Actress Pamela Anderson, musician Marianne Faithful, author Allen Ginsberg, pathologist Dr Jack Kevorkian, stuntman Evel Knievel, business entrepreneur Anita Roddick

Acute hepatitis (symptoms less than 6 months)
Prodrome
- Arthralgia
- Malaise
- Nausea and vomiting

Acute hepatitis signs
- Icterus (scleral)
- Jaundice
- Lymphadenopathy
- Sometimes splenomegaly
- Tender hepatomegaly

Chronic hepatitis (symptoms more than 6 months)
Symptoms of chronic liver disease such as jaundice, cirrhosis, fatigue.

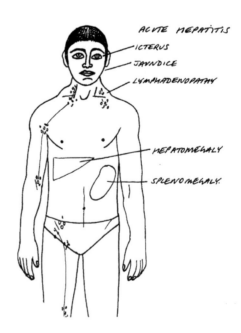

FIGURE 7.15

Hepatomegaly, splenomegaly, hepatosplenomegaly

Hepatomegaly: causes
- Alcoholism
- Carcinoma – primary or secondary
- Right heart failure

Splenomegaly: causes
- Amyloidosis
- Infectious – (**CRIME**):
    C CMV
    R Rheumatic fever
    I Infective endocarditis
    M Malaria
    E Encapsulated bacteria
- Lymphoid – leukaemias and lymphomas
- Sarcoidosis

Hepatosplenomegaly: causes
- Anaemias (sickle cell, pernicious, thalassaemia)
- Autoimmune hepatitis
- Budd–Chiari's
- Chagas' disease
- Cirrhosis
- Endocrine causes (acromegaly, thyroid disease, SLE)
- Infectious (hepatitis, infectious mononucleosis)
- Lymphoid (leukaemias and lymphomas)
- Malaria
- Marrow (polycythaemia vera)
- Portal hypertension
- Spherocytosis
- Toxoplasmosis

Inflammatory bowel disease: ulcerative colitis

Definition
An inflammatory bowel disease that leads to ulcers in the colon, character-ised by exacerbations and remissions.

Well-known people with ulcerative colitis
Sportsperson Sir Steve Redgrave

Ulcerative colitis (ULCERS)
U Ulcers (limited to mucosa and submucosa)
L Large intestine (rectum always involved, may extend proximally to involve entire colon) – non-granulomatous

C CRAMPS (lower abdominal), tenesmus/urgency
E Extra-intestinal manifestations (PS)
    P Pyoderma gangrenosum
    S Sclerosing cholangitis
R Remnants of old ulcers (pseudopolyps), **R**elapsing and **R**emitting pattern
S Stools bloody, may contain mucus and pus

Definition of a severe attack (EAT STEroid)

E ESR >30 mm/h
A Albumin <30 g/L
T Temp at 6.00 a.m. >37.8 °C
S Stool frequency >6 stools per day with blood
T Tachycardia
E anaEmia

Complications of UC

- Cancer
- Toxic megacolon

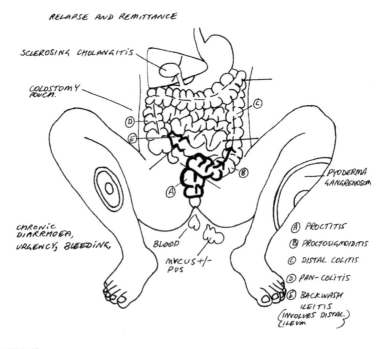

ULCERATIVE COLITIS

RELAPSE AND REMITTANCE

SCLEROSING CHOLANGITIS

COLOSTOMY POUCH.

PYODERMA GANGRENOSUM

CHRONIC DIARRHOEA, URGENCY, BLEEDING,

BLOOD

MUCUS+/- PUS

(A) PROCTITIS
(B) PROCTOSIGMOIDITIS
(C) DISTAL COLITIS
(D) PAN-COLITIS
(E) BACKWASH ILEITIS (INVOLVES DISTAL ILEUM)

FIGURE 7.16

Inflammatory bowel disease: Crohn's disease (granulomatous colitis)

Definition
Inflammatory disease that can affect any part of the gastrointestinal tract.

Well-known people with Crohn's disease
Possibly Alfred the Great, singer Anastacia, actress Shannon Doherty

Crohn's disease
- Abdominal pain (may be mistaken for appendicitis)
- Any portion of GI tract affected, particularly ileocaecal, rectum often spared
- Cobblestone appearance of mucosa
- Granulomas often present
- High temperature
- Iritis

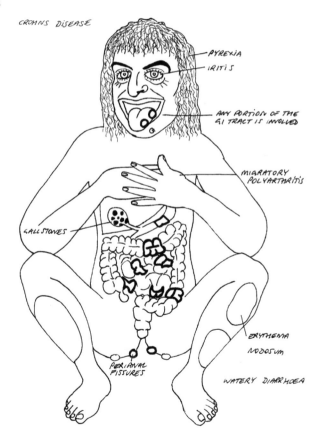

FIGURE 7.17

- Malabsorption
- Mesenteric lymph node hyperplasia
- Perianal fissures, fistulas
- Rose-thorn ulcers
- Skip lesions
- Strictures are common
- Transmural inflammation, thick wall (as apposed to thin wall in UC)
- Watery diarrhoea

Extra-intestinal manifestations of Crohn's disease
- Erythema nodosum
- Gallstones
- Iritis
- Migratory polyarthritis

Complications of Crohn's disease
- Abnormal connections (fistulas/strictures)
- Cancer (rarer than in UC)
- Malabsorption

Indications for surgery (CHOP IT)
C Carcinoma/Connections that are abnormal, i.e. fistulae
H Haemorrhage
O Obstruction
P Perforation
I Infection
T failure to Thrive in children (Crohn's)

Pancreatitis
Well-known people with pancreatitis
Possibly Alexander the Great, composer Ludwig Van Beethoven

Acute pancreatitis
Risk factors for acute pancreatitis (GET SMASHED)
G Gallstones
E Ethanol
T Trauma
S Steroids
M Mumps
A Autoimmune
S Scorpion bites
H Hyperlipidaemia/Hypercalcaemia
E ERCP
D Drugs, azathioprine, diuretics

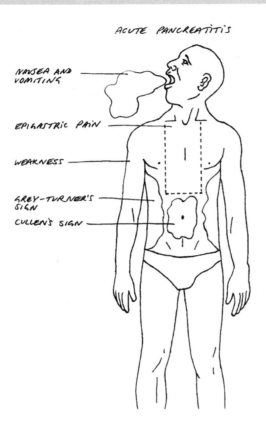

ACUTE PANCREATITIS

NAUSEA AND VOMITING

EPIGASTRIC PAIN

WEAKNESS

GREY-TURNER'S SIGN

CULLEN'S SIGN

FIGURE 7.18

Acute pancreatitis, presentation (NEWTS)

N Nausea and vomiting

E Epigastric pain, severe, radiates to the back

W Weakness

T grey Turner's sign (frank discolouration) and Cullen's sign (periumbilical discolouration) both due to the autodigestion of blood vessels which haemorrhage into the retroperitoneal space, the blood-stained fluid tracks = bruising

S Sepsis may lead to septic shock

Modified Glasgow criteria for predicting severity of pancreatitis (PANCREAS)

P PaO_2 <8 kPa

A Age >55 years

N Neutrophils raised and WCC >15x10⁹/L

C Calcium <2 mmol/L

R Renal function – urea >16 mmol/L

E Enzymes – LDH >600 IU/L, AST >200 IU/L
A Albumin <32 g/L
S Sugar – blood glucose >10 mmol/L

The presence of three or more points within the first 48 hours constitutes severe acute pancreatitis and should warrant transfer to ITU.

Chronic pancreatitis (P-DANCES)
P Persistent epigastric pain, with recurrent episodes
D DM
A Anorexia
N Nausea
C Constipation
E Erythema ab igne (discolouration on front of abdomen due to using a hot water bottle and leaning forward to relieve the discomfort)
S Steatorrhoea

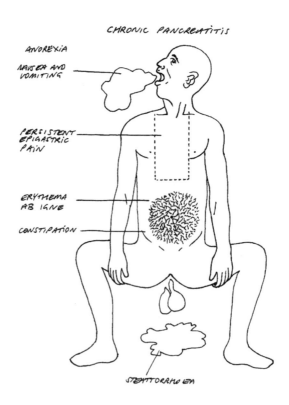

FIGURE 7.19

Portal hypertension

Portal hypertension signs are due to the direct effects of portal hypertension and also the effects of liver cell failure.

Effects of portal hypertension (HOPSCAM)

H **H**aemorrhoids
O **O**esophageal varices can lead to **SCAM**
P **P**eptic ulcers can lead to **SCAM**
S **S**plenomegaly
C **C**aput medusae
A **A**scites
M **M**elaena

Effects of liver cell failure

- Anaemia
- Ankle oedema
- Asterixis, liver flap (coarse hand tremor)
- Bleeding tendency
- Coma
- Foetor hepaticus (breath smells like a corpse)
- Gynaecomastia
- Icterus (scleral)
- Jaundice
- Loss of sexual hair
- Spider naevi
- Testicular atrophy

Renal colic

- Check for hypercalcaemia
- **Bones** (bone pain)
- **Stones** (kidney stones)
- **Groans** (abdominal pain)
- **Psychic moans** (emotional upset, depression, anxiety)
- Bladder stones and haematuria
- Blood pressure is raised
- Constipation
- Corneal calcification
- Enlarged parathyroid glands
- Epigastric pain – groans (abdominal pain)
- Gouty arthritis of feet – bones (bone pain)
- Gouty tophi on ear
- Mental state – moans (emotional upset, depression, anxiety)
- Renal calculi – stones (kidney stones)

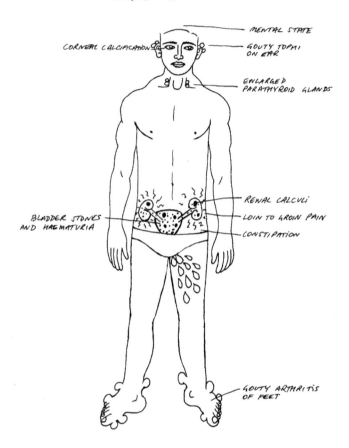

RENAL COLIC

MENTAL STATE

CORNEAL CALCIFICATION

GOUTY TOPHI ON EAR

ENLARGED PARATHYROID GLANDS

RENAL CALCULI

LOIN TO GROIN PAIN

CONSTIPATION

BLADDER STONES AND HAEMATURIA

GOUTY ARTHRITIS OF FEET

FIGURE 7.20

Wilson's disease (3 Cs)

C Ceruloplasmin is decreased

C Copper is excessively deposited in the liver and brain, due to a deficient copper-transporting protein

C Chromosome 13 carries the autosomal recessive defect

Signs and symptoms of Wilson's disease

Children

- Hepatic problems (hepatitis, cirrhosis, fulminant hepatic failure)

Young adults

- Neurological disease (tremor, dysarthria, dyskinesias, dementia)

General signs and symptoms

- Anaemia, haemolytic
- Asterixis (basal ganglia degeneration)
- Kayser–Fleischer's rings in the cornea (green-brown deposits of copper in Descemet's membrane)
- Liver abnormalities (jaundice secondary to hepatitis/cirrhosis, hepatomegaly)
- Neurological symptoms (loss of coordination, tremor, dysphagia, choreiform movements, rigidity)
- Psychiatric symptoms (psychosis, anxiety, mania, depression, dementia)

8

Neurology: cranial nerves

Contents

Neurological history

Refer to the general examination chapter for full history. Note if the patient is left or right handed.

- Balance problems
- Difficulty in talking, chewing or swallowing
- Dizziness or blackouts
- Headaches and visual problems
- Mood changes
- Numbness or pins and needles
- Sensation changes (smell, vision, taste or hearing).

- Sleep disturbance
- Weakness of the limbs or difficulty in mobilising

Neurological examination
Pre-examination checklist (WIPERS)
Inspection
General
A **A**ppearance – glasses, dark glasses, white stick, walking stick, Zimmer frame, facial asymmetry, hearing aids, etc.

B **B**ehaviour – speech abnormalities (dysphasia, dysarthria, dysphonia)

C **C**onnections – NG feed, PEG feed, EEG machine, etc.

Cranial nerve I: olfactory
Ask if they have noticed any change in their sense of smell?

Inspect nasal passages with a torch for obstructions, deviated septum. Occlude one nostril with your finger and check the other one with essence bottles of scent such as coffee, ask them to identify it with their eyes closed. *Usually not tested.*

Cranial nerve II: optic
- Test visual acuity, colour vision, pupillary reflexes, visual fields and fundoscopy
- If the patient usually wears glasses use them. Observe the eyes for abnormalities, *see* Eye abnormalities, p. 90.
- Test each eye separately for acuity (Snellen chart) and colour vision (Ishihara chart). Or ask them to read and identify colours. Examine the pupillary reflexes, *see* Pupillary reflexes, p. 91. Sit opposite the patient and examine the visual fields by confrontation, *see* Visual fields, p. 87. Examine fundi, *see* Opthalmoscopy, p. 89.

Cranial nerves III, IV, VI: oculomotor, trochlear, abducens
- Test the muscles that control pupillary size, eye movement and the muscles that control the upper eyelid.
- Examine pupils – shape, relative size, ptosis.
- Test response to light – ask the patient to stare into the distance, shine light, move in from the side and then straight along the visual axis to provide maximal stimulation, assess the direct and consensual responses.
- Ask the patient to 'Follow my finger with your eyes without moving your head and tell me if you have any double-vision.' Hold your finger approximately 60 cm from the patient and move in an H pattern while looking for limitation of movement/nystagmus/conjugate gaze weakness (upward/lateral) – gaze palsy = supranuclear lesion. Fatiguability (myasthenia)? Strabismus? Normal subjects may exhibit

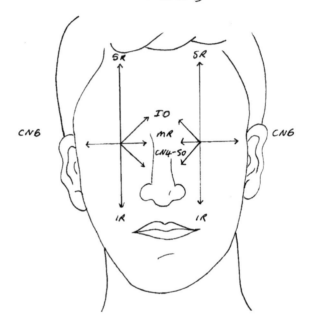

FIGURE 8.1

minor degrees of nystagmus at extremes of lateral gaze. *See* Eye movements, p. 90.

- Test convergence by asking the patient to concentrate on the tip of your finger as you move it towards the bridge of their nose.
- Test accommodation by asking the patient to look into the distance and then at your finger which is held 30 cm from their nose.

Cranial nerve V: trigeminal
Sensation
Compare facial sensation on either side of the face. Test light touch (cotton wool) and pain (sterile sharp object). Test two-point discrimination using callipers, a separation of 3–4 mm can be detected. Test sensation in each division of the trigeminal nerve on one side and then the other side.

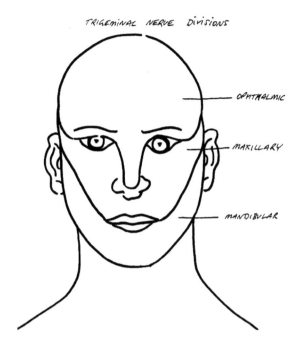

FIGURE 8.2

Corneal reflex is sometimes avoided because it can be uncomfortable – patient looks up and away. Touch the cornea and not the conjunctiva of the eye with a wisp of wet cotton wool. Normal response is for **both** eyes to blink due to contraction of the orbicularis oculi. Repeat on other side – tests V sensory, VII motor.

Motor
Test the motor aspect of V – ask the patient to open their mouth, clench teeth (pterygoids), inspect the muscles of mastication for wasting, palpate the temporal and masseter muscles as they clench. Ask the patient to open their jaw against resistance (pterygoids, mylohyoid, anterior belly of the digastric).

The jaw jerk is sometimes avoided because it can be uncomfortable – place your finger on the tip of the patient's jaw and tap your own finger lightly with a patella hammer. A normal response is for nothing to happen or just a slight closure, often not visible in young people but commonly present in those above the age of 50. An increased jaw jerk occurs due to bilateral diseases of the UMN above the level of the pons (such as pseudobulbar palsy). It is sometimes difficult to distinguish brisk jaw jerk due to pathology or anxiety. *See* Cerebellopontine angle lesion, p. 142 and Cavernous sinus lesion.

Cranial nerve VII facial nerve

Sensation

- Supplies taste sensation to the anterior two-thirds of the tongue (more accurately tested with electrogustometry)
- Supplies parasympathetic secretomotor fibres (via the nervus intermedius) to the lacrimal gland (produces tears) – ophthalmologists test with the Schirmer's test – and submandibular gland (produces saliva) – not usually tested in clinical practice.

Motor

- Inspect for facial droop or asymmetry.
- Ask the patient to look up, wrinkle their forehead, smile, whistle, blow out their cheeks whilst the examiner applies pressure.
- Ask the patient to shut their eyes tightly and try to stop you opening them.

Facial nerve reflexes

The facial nerve is the efferent limb of the corneal reflex (touching the cornea causes contraction of the orbicularis oculi and bilateral blinking), palmomental reflex (scratching the thenar eminence causes contraction of the ipsilateral mentalis muscle), pout or snout reflex (brisk tap on the lips causes bilateral pursing of the lips), nasopalpebral reflex (glabellar tap) and the efferent limb of the stapedius reflex.

See UMNL vs. LMNL (p. 168).

Cranial nerve VIII: vestibulocochlear

This cranial nerve has two parts the vestibular (hearing) and the cochlear (posture, eye coordination and movement).

Hearing

Hearing is better quantified with audiometry and brain-stem evoked potentials. Bedside tests are to see if hearing is normal or abnormal, this involves whispering numbers or words and using Rinne's test. If an abnormality is detected Weber's test is used to detect if it is symmetrical or asymmetrical.

Test hearing

To obstruct hearing in the non-tested ear rustle your fingers together outside the ear or gently massage the external acoustic meatus. Whisper a number or some words into the tested ear and ask the patient to repeat them. This tests for higher frequencies. Compare both sides.

Rinne's test – compares air vs. bone conduction. Normal response is that air conduction (ear) is better than bone conduction (mastoid). Place a 512/1024 Hz vibrating fork on the mastoid bone behind each ear. Ask the patient to say when they stop hearing it. When they stop hearing it, point the prongs at the patient's ear and ask if they can hear it. Complete the examination by examining the external auditory canals, eardrums with an auroscope.

Weber's test – tests for lateralisation. Place a 512/1024 Hz vibrating fork on top of patient's head and ask them where they can hear the sound the loudest? Normal response is midline. *See* Impaired hearing, p. 134.

Vestibular function

Test for the oculocephalic (doll's-eye) reflex, by turning the head and watching the eyes. Both eyes should move in the opposite direction when the head is moved. A negative response is where the eyes are fixed and do not respond when the head is turned. This test is used to determine brain-stem death. Hallpike's test is used to induce positional nystagmus. This test is best omitted if the patient has any neck problems. Support the patient's head and with their eyes open lower it below the edge of the couch and turn the head to one side. Sit the patient up again and turn their head to the other side. Note the response of the eyes to head movement.

The oculovestibular (caloric) reflex

Eye movements are observed after water is poured into the external ear canal. If cool water (approximately 30 °C) is poured into the external canal the patient should develop nystagmus towards the contralateral side. If warm water (approximately 44 °C) is used the patient should develop nystagmus towards the ipsilateral side. These tests are best carried out in a laboratory that can record eye movements, rather than at the bedside.

Cranial nerves IX-X: glossopharyngeal, vagus

The glossopharyngeal and vagus nerves are often examined together because they are closely interrelated.

Glossopharyngeal

Motor

The motor component is small, innervating the stylopharyngeus and sometimes the palatal and upper pharyngeal muscles. Secretomotor parasympathetic supply to the parotid gland.

Sensory

- Eustachian tube and tympanic cavity sensation
- Mucosa of pharynx and tonsillar region sensation
- Posterior third of tongue, taste sensation

Vagus nerve

Sensory

- Dura mater of posterior cranial fossa
- External auditory meatus skin sensation

- Heart, lungs and intestines are related to the vagus nerve via afferent and efferent connections

Motor (U SIC): the gag reflex's motor component!
U **U**pper pharynx muscles
S **S**oft palate muscles
I **I**ntrinsic muscles of larynx
C **C**ricothyroid

The glossopharyngeal and vagus nerve reflexes
- Carotid sinus reflex – massaging the carotid causes slowing of the heart.
- Gag reflex – tactile stimulation of the upper pharynx and tonsils (IX afferent nerves) causes constriction and elevation of the pharynx and palate (X efferent nerves).
- Oculocardiac reflex – massaging the eyeball causes slowing of the heart.

The glossopharyngeal and vagus nerve examination
- Assess the patient's voice – is it hoarse (recurrent laryngeal nerve palsy) or nasal (X disorder)?
- Ask the patient to cough (bovine cough = recurrent laryngeal nerve palsy).
- Ask the patient to puff out their cheeks – is there palatal closure of the nasopharynx or does the air escape from the nose?
- Examine the palate with a torch – the uvula should be central (unilateral lesion = uvula drawn to normal side). Ask the patient to say 'Ah' and look for symmetrical soft palate movement.
- Ask the patient to swallow some water and check for regurgitation.
- The gag reflex is sometimes omitted because it is unpleasant and should only be performed if there is evidence of nerve palsy. It tests the sensory part of IX and motor part of X. Touch the pharynx or tonsil on each side and check for a normal gag response each time. *See* Glossopharyngeal and vagus nerve lesion, p. 135.

Cranial nerve XI: accessory
Motor
- Supplies the sternomastoid and the upper part of the trapezius muscle.
- Stand behind the patient and examine the trapezius for atrophy and asymmetry.
- Ask the patient to shrug their shoulders and keep them raised while you try to push them down – is there any weakness of the trapezius? Ask them to turn their head against resistance, whilst you palpate the sternomastoid muscle on the opposite side. Repeat for the other side. Examine the scapula – weakness of the trapezius causes the vertebral border of the scapula to protrude at the upper part and rotate towards the spine at its

lower border. The shoulder will appear dropped. Isolated weakness of the trapezius can occur if there is damage to branches of the spinal accessory nerve during surgery to the posterior triangle of the neck.

Cranial nerve XII: hypoglossal
Motor
- Motor supply to the tongue muscles.
- Whilst the tongue is in the patient's mouth inspect it for bulk, wasting and fasciculations.
- Ask the patient to stick their tongue out and observe for symmetry of movement and fasciculations. Ask them to move their tongue from side to side. Does the tongue deviate to the side?
- Ask them to return their tongue to their mouth and press it against the inside of their mouth, so that you can press against their cheek and assess strength and bulk.
- Ask them to say 'La la la.' To assess for hypokinesis of tongue movements.
- Complete the examination by examining the neck and cervical spine. *See* Neck and cervical spine, p. 154.

Hypoglossal nerve abnormalities
Unilateral atrophy
Tongue is thinner and more wrinkled on the affected side and deviates to the unaffected side on protrusion.

Bilateral LMN lesions
Fasciculating and wasted tongue (bulbar palsy)

Unilateral UMN lesions
Deviated tongue without fasciculations and wasting (CVA)

Bilateral UMN lesions
- Hypokinetic movement
- Tongue appears small and conical
- Dysarthria and dysphagia (pseudobulbar palsy)

Orofacial dyspraxias
Inability to move the tongue and some of the facial muscles on command (parietal lobe lesions).

Orofacial dyskinesias
Involuntary movements of the tongue and some facial muscles. Often drug induced (antiparkinsonian medication).

Deafness and impaired hearing

Normal hearing
- Normal hearing on both sides
- Rinne's test – air conduction > bone conduction
- Weber's test, the sound is heard in the midline

Conductive hearing (tympanic membrane or ossicular chain)
- Hearing decreased on affected side
- Rinne's test – bone conduction > air conduction
- Weber's test – the sound appears to be arising from the deaf side (because bone conduction is better in the presence of middle ear damage)

Sensorineural deafness (organ of Corti or cochlear nerve)
- Hearing decreased on affected side
- Rinne's test – air conduction > bone conduction
- Weber's test – the sound appears to arise from the better ear

Causes of sensorineural deafness (Deaf BAT)
D Damage to cochlear nerve, organ of Corti
B Bilaterally in older people (presbycusis)
A Acoustic neuroma
T Transverse fracture of petrous temporal bone

Causes of conductive deafness (WOODI) *'deaf as a plank!'*
W Wax in the external canal
O Ossicular chain damage (head injury)
O Otosclerosis (degenerative)
D Damage to tympanic membranes
I Inner ear fluid

Funny turn
Accidental fall (trips and slips)

Attention-seeking behaviour/supratentorial
Especially common in children

Drop attack
Sudden weakness in legs causes falls without warning or loss of consciousness (LOC)

Epilepsy
Condition where generalised or partial seizures lead to impaired consciousness or LOC due to disordered discharge of cerebral neurones.

Syncope
Light-headedness, with feeling of impending LOC or actual LOC caused by reduced cerebral blood flow. *See* Syncope, p. 167.

Vertigo
Rotational sensation (room-spinning) with unsteadiness, caused by dysfunction in vestibular system, either central or peripheral.

Central vertiginous disorders
Affecting the central connections of the vestibular nuclei in the brainstem and their connections with the temporal lobes. Associated with neurological symptoms.
- Benign positional vertigo
- Migraine
- Multiple sclerosis

Peripheral vertiginous disorders (SCAM)
Affecting the peripheral vestibular apparatus of the inner ear and vestibular nerve. Associated with cochlear symptoms (unilateral/bilateral deafness and tinnitus).
S **S**kull fracture
C **C**hronic otitis media
A **A**coustic neuroma
M **M**énière's disease

Glossopharyngeal and vagus nerve lesion
Common causes of glossopharyngeal and vagus nerve lesions
- Bilateral X Progressive bulbar palsy (motor neurone disease), Pseudobulbar palsy (bilateral supranuclear lesions) – strokes, multiple sclerosis. *See* Bulbar palsy vs. pseudobulbar palsy, p. 168.
- Recurrent laryngeal nerve damage, Aortic arch aneurysms, Bronchial carcinoma, Mediastinal lymphoma
- Unilateral damage to CN IX and X (Skull base), Skull base fractures, Skull base neoplasms (including meningioma)

Headaches
Raised intracranial pressure (ICP) headaches (BEND)
B **B**ending makes it worse
E **E**arly morning pain wakes from sleep
N **N**ature is often progressive
D **D**isease unless otherwise proven

	MIGRAINE	TENSION HEADACHE	CLUSTER HEADACHE	NEURALGIA	RAISED ICP	SAH
SITE	UNILATERAL	BAND-LIKE	UNILATERAL, EYE, NOSE, CHEEK	TRIGEMINAL NERVE DISTRIBUTION		OCCIPITAL
ONSET	GRADUAL	GRADUAL			GRADUAL	SUDDEN
CHARACTER	DULL, THROBBING	PRESSURE		PAROXYSMS INTENSE PAIN		THUNDERCLAP
RADIATION		NECK AND SHOULDERS				
ASSOCIATIONS	AURA, NAUSEA + VOMITING, PHOTOPHOBIA	ANXIETY	EYE AND NOSE TEARING		VOMITING OFTEN WITHOUT NAUSEA	NECK STIFFNESS
TIMING	24–72 HOURS	MINUTES–MONTHS	1 HOUR, EARLY MORNING	PAROXYSMS LAST SECONDS	SEVERE PAIN WAKES FROM SLEEPING	
EXACERBATING AND ALLEVIATING FACTORS	CHOCOLATE SEE MNEMONIC PREGNANCY ALLEVIATES	STRESS	SMALL AMOUNTS ALCOHOL (VASODILATOR)	FACIAL MOVEMENT	BENDING COUGHING	
Score on pain scale	10/10			10/10		10/10

Nystagmus
Pendular nystagmus
The amplitude of the two phases of movement is equal

Causes of pendular nystagmus (COP)
- Congenital blindness
- Ocular albinism
- Poor vision

Horizontal phasic (jerk) nystagmus
The direction of horizontal nystagmus is assigned according to the direction of the fast phase, with the fast phase usually being greatest when looking towards the side of the lesion. Horizontal nystagmus is classified into three degrees:

First degree   present only when looking towards the lesion
Second degree   also present when looking straight ahead
Third degree   present even when looking in the opposite direction

Causes of horizontal phasic (jerk) nystagmus
- Brain stem dysfunction
- Cerebellar dysfunction
- Convergence-retraction nystagmus (lesions of tectal and pineal region)
- Downbeat nystagmus (often due to cervicomedullary junction lesions)
- Seesaw nystagmus (parasellar lesions).
- Labyrinthine dysfunction (usually horizontal or rotary)

Causes of multidirectional nystagmus
- Anticonvulsant toxicity
- Brain stem ischaemia
- Multiple sclerosis
- Wernicke's encephalopathy

Mimics of nystagmus
Ocular bobbing
- Spontaneous downward jerks of both eyes and then return to resting position
- Often due to pontine haemorrhage

Opsoclonus
- Chaotic rapid eye movements
- Due to metastatic neuroblastoma in children and bronchogenic carcinoma in adults

Speech disorders

Speech disorders can be divided into three major categories:

- Dysphasia – disorder of language
- Dysarthria – disorder of articulation
- Dysphonia – disorder of phonation, projection of air through larynx

Language areas

Language areas are found in the dominant cerebral hemisphere. Most right-handed people have a dominant left hemisphere. The majority of left-handed people have a left or bilateral language localisation and approximately a third have right dominance.

Broca's area generates motor programmes for word production. Lesion –> reduced vocabulary, poor articulation, non-fluent speech, 'clipped' quality, grammatical errors and of syntax (**BE, IF**):

B Broca's area
E Expressive dysphasia
I Inferior
F Frontal region

Wernicke's area processes the comprehension of language and choosing of words to convey meaning. Lesion –> normal or increased output of speech (like an open water tap), fluent speech, good articulation, but also nonsense words (neologisms), incorrect words (verbal paraphasias) and incorrect letters (literal paraphasias) – literally talking rubbish. (**WateR TAP**):

W Wernicke's area
R Receptive dysphasia
T Temporal
A and Adjoining
P Parietal region

Arcuate fasciculus links Broca's and Wernicke's areas. In conduction dysphasia the arcuate fasciculus of fibres is damaged due to a lesion in the perisylvian area.

Dysphasias

Categories of dysphasias include conductive, receptive, nominal and expressive. The first three are the most common. Ask questions to distinguish between them (**CRN**):

C Command following – tests comprehension of spoken speech. 'Pick up the paper with your right hand, fold it in half and place it on the table'.
R Repeat a statement – detects repetition failure. 'Sunshine makes me happy.'
N Name a shown object.

C Conductive dysphasia
C follow a Command – can do
R Repeat a statement – can **not** do
N Name an object – can **not** do

R Receptive dysphasia
Wernicke's area lesion – cannot understand written or spoken language, speak nonsense
C follow a Command – can **not** do
R Repeat a statement – can **not** do
N Name an object – can **not** do

N Nominal dysphasia
C follow a Command – can do
R Repeat a statement – can do
N Name an object – can **not** do

E Expressive dysphasia
Broca's area lesion – understand language but cannot express themselves in speech or writing
C follow a Command – can do
R Repeat a statement – can **not** do
N Name an object – can **not** do

Dysarthria
Difficulty of articulation – slurs words, cannot say 'British Constitution'
  Causes of dysarthria (**ABCDE**):
A Alcohol (commonest cause)
B Bulbar or pseudobulbar palsy. *See* Bulbar palsy and pseudobulbar palsy, p. 140.
C Cerebellar problems
D Drugs (illicit drugs such as cannabis)
E Extrapyramidal disease such as Parkinson's disease

Dysphonia
Husky voice, low volume – can be caused by recurrent laryngeal nerve palsy, laryngitis

Bell's palsy
Well-known people with Bell's palsy
Actor George Clooney, British comedian Graeme Garden, Indian actor Anupam Kher

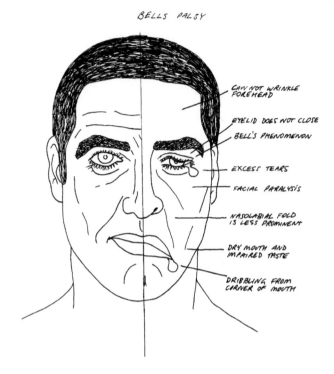

BELLS PALSY

- CAN NOT WRINKLE FOREHEAD
- EYELID DOES NOT CLOSE
- BELL'S PHENOMENON
- EXCESS TEARS
- FACIAL PARALYSIS
- NASOLABIAL FOLD IS LESS PROMINENT
- DRY MOUTH AND IMPAIRED TASTE
- DRIBBLING FROM CORNER OF MOUTH

FIGURE 8.3

Aetiology

Idiopathic but could be due to latent herpes virus reactivation in cranial nerve ganglia – herpes simplex virus type 1 and herpes zoster virus (more aggressive pathology).

Symptoms and signs of Bell's palsy

- Eye watering
- Facial distortion
- Hyperacusis
- Loss of taste
- Lower motor neurone palsy
- Sudden onset facial paralysis
- Usually unilateral
- Wallerian degeneration can follow the initial reversible neurapraxia

Bulbar palsy and pseudobulbar palsy

Bulbar palsy (LAST FIB): *you won't be lying again*

L Lower motor neurone signs

A Absent jaw jerk, or can be normal

S Speech is quiet, hoarse or nasal
T Tongue is flaccid and fasciculating (like a sack of worms)
F Facial muscles are affected
I Involves tongue and muscles of chewing/swallowing
B Brainstem motor nuclei not functioning

Pseudobulbar palsy (AMUSED): *labile emotions*
A Affects muscles of eating, swallowing and talking
M More common than bulbar palsy
U Upper motor neurone lesion
S Strokes affecting corticobulbar pathways bilaterally, MS and MND are common causes
E Emotions may be labile (appear amused and giggle during examination)
D Donald Duck speech due to spastic tongue

Cavernous sinus syndrome
Anatomy of the cavernous sinuses
The cavernous sinuses are twinned venous structures on either side of the sella turcica. The cavernous sinus contains:

- Carotid artery and its sympathetic plexus (pass through the sinus itself)
- Ocular motor nerves III, IV, VI, (pass through the wall of the sinus)
- Trigeminal nerve (ophthalmic branch and occasionally the maxillary branch)

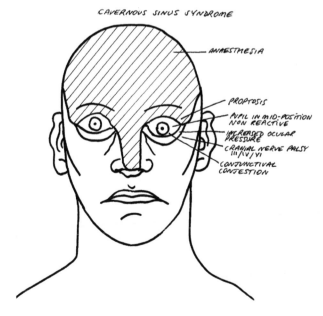

FIGURE 8.4

Causes of cavernous sinus syndrome
- Carotid–cavernous fistulas (C–C fistulas)
- Carotid artery aneurysms
- Neoplasia

Symptoms of cavernous sinus syndrome
Cavernous sinus syndrome affects cranial nerves III, IV, VI and the ophthalmic branch and occasionally maxillary branch of V. Symptoms tend to be unilateral but can be bilateral in neoplasia.

Examination of cavernous sinus syndrome
- Anaesthesia in the ophthalmic division of the trigeminal nerve (V1) with possible decreased or absent corneal reflex. Possibly anaesthesia/paraesthesia in the maxillary or V2 branch.
- Conjunctival congestion
- Cranial nerve palsy III, IV, VI
- Ocular pressure is raised
- Optic disc oedema or pallor
- Ophthalmoplegia (may be painful)
- Proptosis, a pulsating exophthalmos suggests a direct C–C fistula
- Pupil is in the midposition and non-reactive if both sympathetics and parasympathetics from the third nerve are affected

Cerebellopontine angle lesions
Definition
The cerebellopontine angle is situated between the cerebellum and the pons. It is a common site for the growth of acoustic neuromas and leads to a neurological syndrome.

Causes of cerebellopontine angle lesions
- Acoustic neuroma – the most common cause
- Meningioma
- Metastasis

Signs of cerebellopontine angle lesions
- Ataxia and other cerebellar signs
- Cranial nerve palsy VII, VIII (sometimes V and rarely IX)
- Hearing on ipsilateral side is affected, deafness, tinnitus
- Nystagmus, cerebellar jerk nystagmus with the fast phase to the affected side, or vestibular nystagmus with the fast phase to the unaffected side
- Trigeminal nerve function is impaired – motor, sensory and reflexes. Initially it may affect only the corneal reflex, and later the jaw jerk.

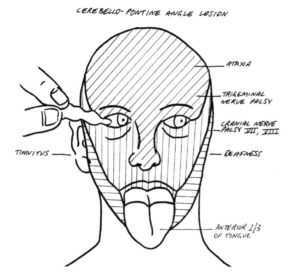

CEREBELLO-PONTINE ANGLE LESION

ATAXIA

TRIGEMINAL NERVE PALSY

CRANIAL NERVE PALSY VII, VIII

TINNITUS

DEAFNESS

ANTERIOR 2/3 OF TONGUE

FIGURE 8.5

Cerebral lesions
Frontal lobe
- Emotional response (antisocial behaviour)
- Personality (loss of inhibition)
- Social behaviour (antisocial behaviour)

Parietal lobe
Dominant side (CLAP)
C Calculation (dyscalculia)
L Language (dysphasia, dyslexia)
A Appreciation of size (apraxia)
P Planned-movement-like clapping (apraxia)

Non-dominant side (SOCS)
Spatial **O**rientation and **C**onstructional **S**kills (neglect of non-dominant side, spatial disorientation, constructional apraxia, dressing apraxia, homonymous hemianopia)

Occipital lobe
Visual analysis – homonymous hemianopia, hemianopic scotomas, visual agnosia, prosopagnosia (poor facial recognition), visual hallucinations (lights, zigzags, lines)

143

Temporal lobe
Dominant side
- Auditory perception – complex hallucinations (smell, sound, vision, homonymous hemianopia)
- Smell – anosmia
- Speech, language – dyslexia, dysphasia
- Verbal memory – poor memory

Non-dominant side
- Auditory perception – complex hallucinations (smell, sound, vision, homonymous hemianopia)
- Music – loss of musical skills
- Non-verbal memory – music, faces, shapes (poor non-verbal memory)
- Smell – anosmia

Language areas
Broca's area and Wernicke's area. *See* speech disorders, p. 138.

Epilepsy
Generalised seizures
Disordered discharge of cerebral neurones involving both hemispheres:
- Absence attacks (petit mal)
- Atonic/Akinetic seizures
- Myoclonic seizures (myoclonic jerks)
- Tonic seizures
- Tonic–clonic seizures (grand mal)

Partial (focal) seizures
Disordered discharge of cerebral neurones from a small area of the cerebral cortex. Temporal lobe epilepsy may lead to olfactory auras and a sensation of déjà vu. Both simple and complex partial seizures can evolve to become generalised seizures.
- Complex partial seizures (LOC)
- Evolving seizures – partial, evolving into generalised seizures
- Generalised seizures with only EEG evidence of focal onset
- Simple partial seizures (no LOC)

Pseudoseizures, non-epileptic attacks
- Attention-seeking behaviour
- Psychosomatic, somatoform disorder
- Supratentorial

Jugular foramen syndrome (Vernet's syndrome)
Definition
The jugular foramen is a large opening in the base of the skull. Jugular foramen syndrome is characterised by the paresis of cranial nerves IX–X1, sometimes with cranial nerve XII.

Causes of jugular foramen syndrome
Basilar skull fracture, tumour

Jugular foramen syndrome
Affects cranial nerves IX, X, XI (and sometimes XII)

IX and X
Features can be divided into motor and sensory

Motor signs
- Articulation – dysarthria, hoarse voice
- Dysphagia with paresis of soft palate, uvula, pharynx and larynx – nasal regurgitation
- Dysphonia – palatal droop on the affected side with ipsilateral vocal cord paralysis and resulting dysphonia
- Sensory signs
- Absence of taste on the posterior third of the tongue
- Depressed gag reflex
- Neuralgic pain in X and IX distribution

XI
Ipsilateral trapezius and sternomastoid muscle weakness and atrophy

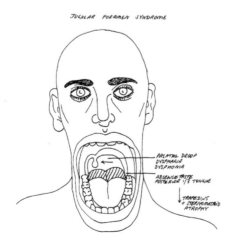

FIGURE 8.6

145

9

Neurology: peripheral nerves

Contents

Neurological examination
Pre-examination checklist (WIPERS)
Inspection
General (ABC)

A Appearance – conscious, decreased consciousness (if so quantify the GCS – refer to Glasgow coma scale), propped up on pillows (need support), hoist, wheelchair, walker, ventilator, syndromic facies – Down's syndrome, Parkinson's disease (mask-like), facial droop (hemiplegia) – visible scars of previous operations, trauma, injury, etc.

B Behaviour – tremor, chorea, athetoid, photophobia (migraine), photophobia and neck stiffness (meningitis), etc.

C Connections – NG tube or PEG (unsafe to swallow), hearing aid (deafness), glasses, medications (anticonvulsants, steroids, anticoagulants, antiparkinsonian drugs, alcohol detoxification regime), etc.

A full nervous examination includes cranial nerves and examination of upper and lower limbs. In this book cranial nerves are treated as a separate chapter.

The upper and lower limbs are examined similarly, compare the right and left sides before testing the next mode, tone is tested before power because movements can increase tone; after you have stood the patient up test gait before sitting them down.

I	Inspection	Neurological system
Tickle	Tone	Motor
Patients	Power	Motor
Get	Gait	Motor
Really	Reflexes	Motor
Cool	Coordination	Sensory
Smiles	Sensation	Sensory

Upper limbs

Inspect (PAID)

P Pronator drift test – ask the patient to close their eyes, arms extended, with palms up. Do the arms drift downward? (UMNL, cerebellar, posterior column loss)

A Asymmetry of muscles and muscle bulk – look for muscle wasting, fasciculations. *See* Motor dysfunction, p. 158.

I Intention tremor (cerebellar), pill-rolling resting tremor (Parkinson's), action tremor (BAT: Benign essential tremor syndrome, Anxiety, Thyrotoxicosis). *See* Involuntary movements, p. 157.

D Deformities – wrist drop, waiter's tip, claw hand

Tone
Ask the patient to relax their muscles and go floppy.

Passively flex and extend each joint in turn slowly at first and then faster to feel for muscle tension. Joints of the upper limb that should be tested are shoulder, elbow joint and wrist joint. Shake hands with the patient whilst supporting the elbow, rotate the two joints to assess resistance. Parkinson's presents with cogwheel rigidity in the wrist (a combination of tremor and increased tone) and lead-pipe resistance on flexing the forearm.

Power
Muscle power is relative to the individual. Muscle power can be assessed with isometric testing (patient contracts a group of muscles as powerfully as possible and maintains the position whilst the examiner tries to overpower the muscle group being tested) or isotonic testing (patient puts joint through a range of movement while the examiner tries to stop the movement progression). Muscle power is quantified using the MRC power scale. *See* MRC power scale, p. 158.

Always ask if there is any tenderness before touching the patient. Try to use the same commands throughout such as 'Don't let me move you.' or 'Pull me towards you, push me away.' Also, ask them to use all of their strength. Assess across a single joint at a time moving in a proximal to distal direction.

The upper limb sequence
- Shoulder AB-duction and AD-duction
- Shoulder flexion and extension
- Elbow flexion and extension
- Wrist flexion and extension
- Forearm supination and pronation
- Finger extension at both the metacarpophalangeal (MCPs) and interphalangeal joints
- Finger and thumb flexion, extension, AB-duction and AD-duction

The abdominal muscles
Ask the patient to lie back and flex their neck to contract their abdominal muscles.

Reflexes
A neurological reflex depends on a reflex arc. Strike the tendon and not the muscle belly in order to activate the reflex arc. Ensure the patient is comfortable and relaxed and that the muscle which is being tested is visible. Compare with the response on the other side. Deep tendon reflexes are classified as:
- Pathologically brisk (clonus)   (++++)
- Hyperactive   (+++)

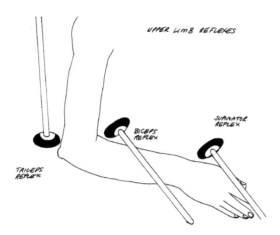

FIGURE 9.1

- Normal   (++)
- Sluggish   (+)
- Absent   (-)
- Biceps   (C5–6)
- Supinator/Brachioradialis   (C5–6)
- Triceps   (C7–8)
- See Deep tendon reflexes, p. 161.

Coordination

Coordination is dependent on the cerebellum. The cerebellum is divided into midline vermis and lateral cerebellar hemispheres. The vermis helps maintain posture, the trunk and gait. The cerebellar hemispheres control limb movement on the ipsilateral side. *See* Cerebellar disorders, p. 168.

Finger-nose test

Ask the patient to repeatedly touch your finger and then their own nose as quickly as possible. Test with the other arm. Move your fingertip so that it is a moving target. To test for sensory ataxia ask the patient to close their eyes and stretch their arm out and then touch the tip of their own nose. Past-pointing (dysmetria) with an intention tremor, generalised clumsiness (dyssynergia) indicates a cerebellar hemisphere lesion.

Rapid alternating movement

Ask the patient to place the palm of their dominant hand on the palm of the opposite hand and then repeatedly flip their dominant hand quickly; repeat with the other hand – dysdiadochokinesia (slowness and incoordination on performing rapid alternating movement)

Sensory

The sensory modalities are pain, temperature, proprioception (joint position sense), and vibration sense.

The modalities tested clinically are:

- **Light touch** Dorsal columns, medial lemniscus
- **Proprioception (joint position sense)** via large fast-conducting axons
- **Two-point discrimination**
- **Vibration sense**
- **Pin prick** Spinothalamic tracts
- **Temperature** slower-conducting axons
- **Stereognosis** Parietal cortex
- **Graphaesthesia**

If there is peripheral sensory loss, try to establish a sensory level. *See* Spinal cord lesions, p. 163.

Pain and temperature (spinothalamic tracts)

Ask the patient to close their eyes and say 'Yes' when they can feel you touching them. Dab the skin alternatively with a sharp and then a blunt instrument such as a sterile toothpick and tongue-depressor and ask them to say whether it was sharp or dull. Test each dermatome. (Testing for deep pain is often avoided.) Deep pain is elicited by squeezing muscle bellies or by pressing down on the finger- and toenails. Temperature can be tested using a cold object such as a tuning fork. Alternatively fill two cups, one with cold water and one with warm water and ask the patient to distinguish between the two.

Light touch (dorsal columns)

Ask the patient to close their eyes and say 'Yes' when they can feel you touching them. Dab the skin lightly with cotton wool, do not stroke. Compare the upper limbs with each other.

Vibration sense (dorsal columns)

Use a 128 Hz tuning fork and once vibrating place it on the patient's sternum so they know what buzzing feels like. Ask the patient to close their eyes and place the tuning fork on their interphalangeal joint of the forefinger. Ask them to say 'Yes' when they can feel the buzzing sensation and 'Now' when the buzzing stops. Stop the tuning fork and see if they respond correctly. If their vibration sense is poor assess the bony prominences moving more peripherally, metacarpophalangeal joint > wrist joint > elbow joint > shoulder joint, both anterior and posterior. *See* Dermatomes, p.154.

Proprioception/joint position sense (dorsal columns)

Begin distally and move more peripherally. Hold the patient's distal phalanx from the sides, avoiding the nail bed, move it up and down and ask the patient to respond 'Up' and 'Down' appropriately. Ask the patient to close their eyes and move their distal phalanx up and down and then leave it in one of those positions and ask the patient to correctly identify its position. If they are unable to do so move more proximally, distal interphalangeal (DIP) joint –> proximal interphalangeal (PIP) joint –> metacarpophalangeal (MCP) joint –> wrist –> elbow.

Two-point discrimination
If a two-point discriminator is not available improvise with a paper clip. Ask the patient to close their eyes. Whilst holding the patient's hands ask them to correctly identify if it is one or two points you are holding against the pulp of their index finger. Determine the minimum distance at which two points can be discriminated, normally 3–5 mm.

Further tests for Point localisation
Ask the patient to close their eyes and identify where you are touching them on their body. Inability could be due to lesions in the posterior inferior parietal cortex.

Stereognosis
Ask the patient to close their eyes and place various easily identifiable objects in their palm and ask them to identify them by sensation alone. The inability to perform this task (astereognosis) could indicate an abnormality of the angular and supramarginal gyri of the parietal lobe.

Graphaesthesia
Ask the patient to close their eyes and with a blunt object trace letters on their palm and ask them to identify the letters. The inability to perform this task (dysgraphaesthesia) suggests an abnormality in the parietal sensory association cortex.

Sensory inattention
Ask the patient to close their eyes and stretch out their arms; touch one or both hands and ask the patient to indicate if it was one side or the other or both.

Abnormal sensations (PAND)
P Pain, noxious symptom
A Altered sensations, paraesthesiae (spontaneous) or dysaesthesiae elicited by other stimuli)
N Numbness
D Decreased sensation (hypoaesthesia)

Lower limbs

Inspect (BAD)

B Bruised, injured and infected feet from peripheral neuropathy

A Asymmetry of muscles and muscle bulk, look for muscle wasting, fasciculations

D Deformities: claw foot (Charcot–Marie–Tooth), clubbed feet

Tone

The lower limb examination for tone is easier than the upper limb equivalent. Simply roll the leg internally and externally and feel for resistance. Also quickly lift the leg off the bed and observe whether the ankle is also raised off the bed. *See* Motor dysfunction, p. 158.

Power

- Hip flexion and extension, AB-duction and AD-duction
- Knee flexion and extension
- Foot dorsiflexion, plantar flexion, inversion and eversion, toe plantar flexion and dorsiflexion. *See* MRC power scale, p. 158.

Gait

Ensure that the patient is safe to mobilise by themselves, they should use a mobility aide if needed. It may be necessary to walk close to them to catch them should they fall. Watch how they get up from a seated position – is there difficulty initiating movement (Parkinson's disease), are they unable to get up without using their arms (proximal myopathy).

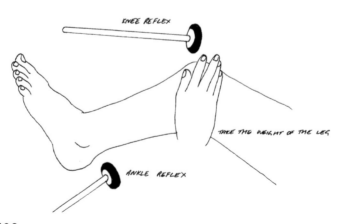

FIGURE 9.2

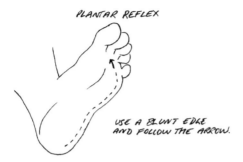

PLANTAR REFLEX

USE A BLUNT EDGE
AND FOLLOW THE ARROW.

FIGURE 9.3

Additional gait tests

Walk heel to toe – diminished ability in midline cerebellar problems. Walk on heels – diminished ability in L4–5 foot-drop.

Ask the patient to stand and then close their eyes – they are Romberg's sign positive if unsteadiness is worse when their eyes are closed.

Reflexes

- Knee (L3–4)
- Ankle (S1–2)
- Plantar (L5, S1–2)
- Test for ankle clonus – bend the patient's knee with the thigh externally rotated. Lift the patient's heel and quickly dorsiflex the ankle – hold it flexed for 3 seconds. It is classified as clonus if sustained movement occurs afterwards.

See Deep tendon reflexes, p. 161.

Coordination

Heel-shin test – ask the patient to place the heel of their right foot on the knee of their left leg and slide it down the shin, and then kick out their right foot to touch your hand before placing their foot on the knee again. Repeat quickly and as smoothly as possible. Repeat with the other foot.

Sensory

Test all dermatomes with all sensation modalities as with the upper limb examination. If peripheral sensory loss, try to establish sensory level. Examine sensation in saddle region, test anal reflex (S2–4).

Vibration sense

Often lost at the ankles over the age of 70, but also an important and early feature of peripheral neuropathy.

Proprioception/joint position sense (dorsal columns)

Start at the interphalangeal joint of the big toe – if there is an impairment move proximally, metatarsophalangeal joint –> ankle joint –> knee joint. Proprioception is first assessed peripherally. *See* Dermatomes, p. 154.

Complete the examination

Assess the spine for deformity (scoliosis, kyphosis), scars (injury, operations), neurofibromas. Gently palpate for tenderness over vertebral bodies (metastatic disease can be very tender).

Test straight-leg raising – ask the patient to try to lift their straight leg – full lifting will be prevented if there is a slipped disc.

Cervical spine and neck

Cervical spine

Test passive and active movements.

Lhermitte's sign

Electric-shock-like pain that runs down the back and limbs triggered by flexing the neck. MS, syringomyelia, spondylotic myelopathy, cervical cord tumours.

Neck

Test for neck stiffness and meningeal irritation.

Inflamed meninges become irritated and cause spasm of the paravertebral muscles causing neck stiffness.

Brudzinski's sign

Ask the patient to lie flat with head supported on a single pillow.

Take the occiput in your hands and gently flex the neck until the chin touches the chest (Brudzinski's sign) or as tolerated by the patient.

Kernig's test

Ask the patient to lie flat with both legs exposed and passively flex one leg at both the knee and hip. Now extend the knee whilst its hip is still flexed. Kernig's positive occurs when the attempt to extend the knee is resisted by the hamstrings and the other leg may flex at the hip.

Dermatomes

An approximate guide to root and area:

C4 – shoulder tip
C5 – outer part of the upper arm
C6 – lateral aspect of the forearm and the thumb
C7 – middle finger (flipping the bird!)
C8 – little finger

T1 – medial aspect of the upper arm
T7 – xiphisternum
T10 – level of umbilicus
L2 – upper thigh
L3 – around the knees
L4 – medial aspect of the leg
L5 – lateral aspect of the leg, medial side of the dorsum of the foot
S1 – lateral aspect of the foot, the heel and most of the sole

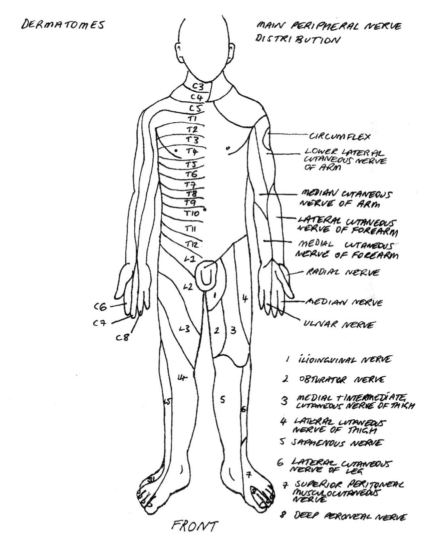

FIGURE 9.4A

S2 – posterior aspect of the thigh
S3, S4, S5 – concentric rings around the anus

Gait abnormalities

- Antalgic gait (OA/joint pain or soft tissue injury) – compensate by leaning on other leg
- Apraxic gait (hydrocephalus/multi-infarct states). Patient has broad-

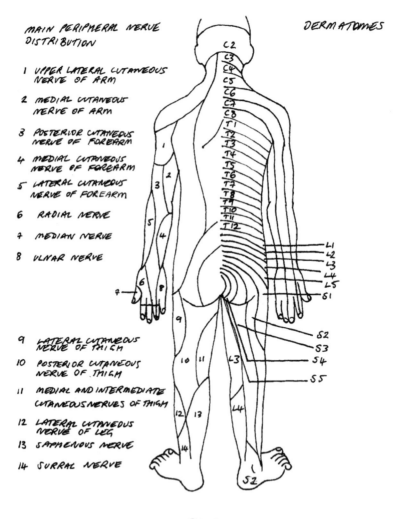

BACK

FIGURE 9.4B

based unsteady gait and takes small steps. Has difficulty in navigating corners.

- Cerebellar (ataxic) broad-based gait. May sway from side to side and need to hold on to objects for support.
- Hemiplegic gait – swinging one leg in a lateral arc (hemiplegia secondary to stroke/cerebral palsy). Hemiparesis – the patient drags affected leg stiffly, foot inverted, arm flexed at the side.
- High-stepping gait (foot drop) – the hip is flexed, the foot is lifted off the ground and then dropped.
- Normal gait
- Parkinsonian (festinating) gait – slow to initiate movement, small steps (festinating gait). Once initiated may walk faster but may have difficulty turning corners or may suddenly freeze. There is a lack of arm-swinging and poverty of postural reflexes and may lean forward and have a tendency to fall over.
- Spastic gait (UMNL) – bilateral spastic gait, patient leans forward, legs are AD-ducted, walks stiffly on toes (equinus).
- Trendelenberg's gait (proximal myopathy)
- Waddling gait, proximal myopathy
- Involuntary movements

Athetosis
Slow, writhing, snake-like movements of fingers and toes

Choreiform movements
Rapid jerking, semi-purposeful and not sustained. Classically seen in Huntington's chorea.

Dystonic movements
Slow sustained writhing movements can lead to sustained abnormal contracture and limb posturing. Often due to basal ganglia pathology.

Hemiballismus
Continuous flailing of arm or leg on one side. Can be violent. Caused by cerebrovascular disease involving the subthalamic nucleus.

Myoclonus
Sudden shock-like movements without purpose, can affect muscles, groups of muscles or the whole body. May occur in normal people when falling asleep.

Causes of myoclonus (SACS): *time to hit the sack!*
S Sleeping (falling asleep)
A Anoxic cerebral brain damage

C Creutzfeldt–Jakob's disease
S Subacute sclerosing panencephalitis

Orofacial-lingual dyskinesias
Chewing, grimacing, affects face, mouth and tongue.

Tics (habit spasms)
Repetitive jerking, more localised and stereotyped than choreiform movements, and can be temporarily resisted by patients. Can affect the respiratory muscles and the voice.

Tremor
Rhythmical movement resulting from the alternating contraction and relaxation of a group of muscles. Produces oscillations about a joint or group of joints. Can affect the whole body.

Types of tremors (PRIK)
P Physiological tremor – rapid and of fine amplitude
R Resting tremor – pill-rolling tremor with the thumb moving across the tips of the other fingers, reduced by voluntary movement
I Intention tremor – absent at rest, apparent on actively holding a position, and made worse by movement
K Kinetic (action) tremor – coarser tremor, on active movement and disappear at rest. Seen in multiple sclerosis, cerebrovascular disease involving midbrain red nucleus ('rubral-type' tremor)

Medical Research Council (MRC) power scale
0 No movement
1 Twitch but no movement of joint
2 Movement, but not against gravity
3 Movement against gravity, but not resistance
4 Movement against resistance, but not entirely normal
5 Normal

Motor dysfunction
- Atrophy – is seen in LMNL and myopathies.
- Fasciculations – subcutaneous twitches overlying muscle bellies when the muscles are at rest. May be coarse or fine and are more commonly found in wasted muscles.
- Impaired coordination
- Involuntary movements (dyskinesias)
- Loss of learned movement patterns
- Paralysis or weakness
- Rate of movement changes (hypokinesia and bradykinesia)

- Tone and posture changes (clonus, rigidity, increased tone and hypotonia, spasticity). Tone can be described as the resistance felt when a joint is moved passively through its range of movement.

Fasciculations
Causes of fasciculations
- Exercise in normal people
- LMN disease that causes a brief contraction of single motor units
- Myokymia, fasciculations of the orbicularis oculi caused by tiredness and anxiety

Abnormal tone
- Clonus – a rhythmic series of involuntary muscle contractions evoked by sudden stretch of muscles. Ankle clonus can be elicited by sustained pressure on the foot and leads to rhythmical alternation of plantar and dorsiflexion. A few beats of clonus are not pathological but sustained clonus indicates an UMNL. Knee clonus can also be elicited by pushing the patella towards the foot sharply while the patient lies supine with the knee extended. Following the initial jerk sustained pressure is applied to the patella in a downwards direction.
- Increased tone (hypertonia) – indicates an UMN lesion.
- Decreased tone (hypotonia) – hypotonia indicates LMN lesion, cerebellar disorders and chorea.
- Rigidity – the sustained resistance to passive movement. Most often seen in Parkinson's disease, it may be 'cogwheel rigidity' where it is phasic and jerky, or sustained through the range of movement.
- Spasticity – rapid build-up of resistance during the first few degrees of passive movement which then gives way to a sudden lessening of resistance. In the upper limb it is more obvious on extension; in the lower limb it is more obvious on flexion.

Nerve roots
A myotome is a group of muscles innervated by a specific spinal segment.
C4 – spontaneous breathing (C4–C5 keep the diaphragm alive)
C5 – shoulder shrug, deltoid
C6 – biceps, brachioradialis, wrist extension
C7 – triceps, ulnar extensors of wrist, wrist flexion
C8 – finger flexors
T1–T12 – intercostals, abdominals
L1/L2 – hip flexion
L3/L4 – hip adduction, quadriceps
L5 – extensor hallucis longus, big toe dorsiflexion
S1/S2 – foot plantarflexion
S2–S4 – rectal tone

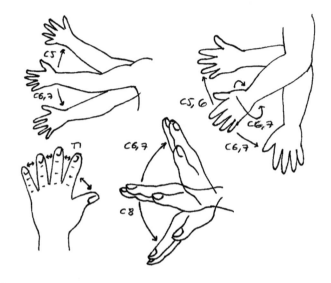

FIGURE 9.5

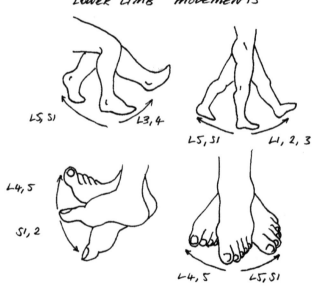

FIGURE 9.6

Reflexes
Deep tendon reflexes
- Reflex reinforcement techniques
- Patient clasps hands together tightly, and releases them just before the tap, (Jendrassik's manoeuvre)
- Patient clasps object tightly
- Patient clenches teeth together – when testing upper limbs

Upper limb reflexes
- Biceps (C5–6)
- Supinator/brachioradialis (C5–6)
- Triceps (C7–8)
- Fingers (C7-T1)

Biceps (C5–6)
Ask the patient to relax their arm and place the elbow at 90 degrees.
 Place your finger over the biceps tendon and allow the tendon hammer to fall on your finger under gravity.

Supinator/brachioradialis (C5–6)
Ask the patient to relax their arm and place the elbow at 90 degrees.
 Keep the hand pronated and allow the tendon hammer to fall under gravity on the distal end of radius.

Triceps (C7–8)
Ask the patient to relax their arm and cross it over their chest.
 Hold the tendon hammer vertically and swing the mallet gently at the triceps tendon.

Fingers (C7-T1)
Ask the patient to relax their hand with the palm up, fingers slightly flexed.
 Place your hand on top of the patient's, pads overlying pads, and gently tap your own fingers.

Lower limb reflexes
- Knees (L3–4)
- Ankles (S1–2)
- Plantars (L5, S1–2)

Knees (L3–4)
With the patient supine, ask the patient to relax their legs and lift both knees with one arm, flexing the legs slightly. The tendon hammer falls with gravity on to the patellar tendon.
 Alternatively, examine in the seated position – ask the patient to cross

their legs and holding the tendon hammer vertically allow the mallet to swing against patellar tendon.

Ankles (S1–2)
With the patient supine, ask the patient to relax their feet, Hold patient's foot so that the ankle and knee joint are at 90 degrees. Gently tap the Achilles tendon.

Plantars (L5, S1–2)
Inform the patient that you are going to rub the sole of their foot and that it might be ticklish or uncomfortable. It is more hygienic to use a disposable orange stick rather than a key. Use the orange stick to stroke from heel, up lateral sole, then medially across to ball of foot. Watch the big toe, normal response is for it to go down, if it goes up this indicates an (UMNL).

See UMNL vs. LMNL, p. 168.

Other deep tendon reflexes include:
Deltoid reflex (C5)
Place your finger on the deltoid muscle belly (on the tip of the shoulder) and tap with the tendon hammer.

Pectoral reflex (C7)
Place your index and middle finger on the lateral border of the pectoralis muscle and tap with a tendon hammer.

Finger jerk (C7-T1)
Place the tips of your middle and index fingers across the palmar surface of the proximal phalanges of the patient's fingers and tap gently. A normal response is slight flexion, and is more pronounced in hyperreflexia.

Hoffmann's reflex (C7, C8, T1)
Place your right index finger under the distal interphalangeal (DIP) of the patient's middle finger and flick the tip down with your thumb, watch the patients thumb for movement. Reflex flexion is increased in hyperreflexia.

Hamstring jerk (L5, S1)
Abnormal deep tendon reflexes
Hyperreflexia and hyporeflexia are signs of UMNL and LMNL respectively. Other abnormal deep tendon reflexes are:
- Anterior horn cell lesions (polio, MND) will lead to decreased/absent deep tendon reflexes.
- Crossed reflex induction refers to excitation of a deep tendon reflex on one side leading to a reflex response on the other side.
- Elderly people may lose or markedly lessen their ankle jerks

- Holmes–Adie's syndrome involves patients with myotonic pupils having some of their deep tendon reflexes absent.
- Peripheral neuropathy may lead to a symmetrical loss of reflexes.
- Radiculopathy affecting a segment may lead to an isolated loss of a reflex (biceps jerk lost with C5–6 disc prolapse, triceps jerk lost with C6–7 prolapse, loss of ankle jerk with S1 disc prolapse).

Superficial tendon reflexes
The superficial tendon reflexes are polysynaptic reflexes that are elicited by cutaneous stimulation.

Plantar response
Strong tactile stimulation of the lateral border of the sole of the foot causes the toe to be down-going and AD-duction of the other toes. Babinski's response – up-going big toe indicates UMNL.

Superficial abdominal reflex
Light tactile stimulation of the abdominal wall causes reflex contraction of the anterior abdominal wall. The umbilicus will move towards the quadrant that is stimulated.

Cremasteric reflex
Stimulation of the male thigh causes the retraction of the ipsilateral testicle, this reflex is dependent on the genitofemoral nerve (L1, L2).

Primitive reflexes (MPRAGS)
The primitive reflexes are present in neonates but disappear in normal adults.
M Moro
P Placing
R Rooting
A Atonic neck reflex
G Grasping
S Snout and pout reflex

Spinal cord lesions (ABCD)
A Anterior spinal artery syndrome – dorsal column function is preserved with loss of spinothalamic function and motor function.
B Brown–Séquard's syndrome – ipsilateral loss of motor function, vibration and JPS and contralateral loss of spinothalamic sensation.
C Cauda equina syndrome (central disc prolapse, metastatic neoplasia, neurofibroma). Sensory loss involving genitalia, perineum, buttocks, back of legs, feet.
  C Central cord syndrome, shawl distribution pain and temperature loss.

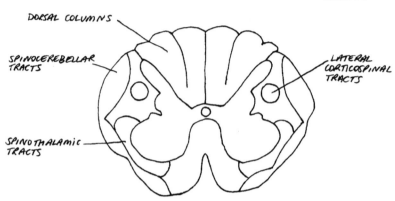

FIGURE 9.7

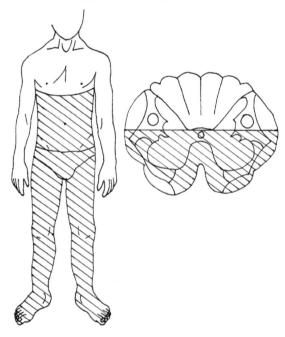

FIGURE 9.8

BROWN-SEQUARD SYNDROME
(UNILATERAL HEMI-CORD LESION)

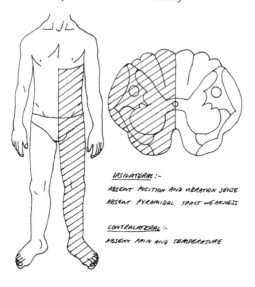

IPSILATERAL:-
ABSENT POSITION AND VIBRATION SENSE
ABSENT PYRAMIDAL TRACT WEAKNESS

CONTRALATERAL:-
ABSENT PAIN AND TEMPERATURE

FIGURE 9.9

CENTRAL CORD SYNDROME

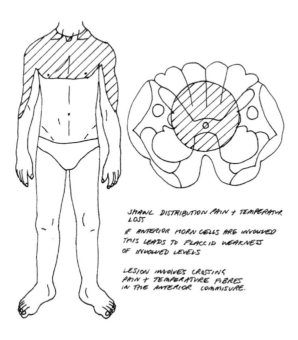

SHAWL DISTRIBUTION PAIN + TEMPERATURE
LOSS
IF ANTERIOR HORN CELLS ARE INVOLVED
THIS LEADS TO FLACCID WEARNESS
OF INVOLVED LEVELS

LESION INVOLVES CROSSING
PAIN + TEMPERATURE FIBRES
IN THE ANTERIOR COMMISURE.

FIGURE 9.10

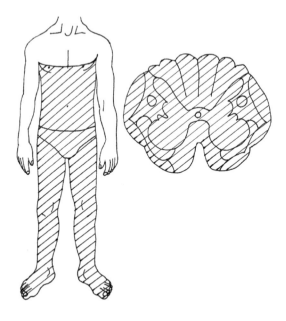

COMPLETE CORD TRANSECTION

FIGURE 9.11

   C Complete cord transaction.
D Dissociated sensory loss (not all modalities are affected equally) involves loss of pain and temperature sensations leaving touch, vibration and JPS unaffected. This is due to damage to the lateral spinothalamic pathways but not the dorsal columns. This is pathognomonic for cervical syringomyelia.

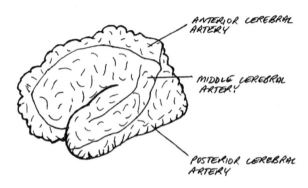

CEREBRAL ARTERY TERRITORIES

ANTERIOR CEREBRAL ARTERY

MIDDLE CEREBRAL ARTERY

POSTERIOR CEREBRAL ARTERY

FIGURE 9.12

Strokes and their arterial territories

MAIN ARTERY	BRANCH	CLINICAL FEATURES	SIDE
Internal carotid	**Middle cerebral artery (MCA)**	Hemiparesis (face+arm > leg) Hemianopia Hemianaesthesia Dysphasia Dysarthria Dyspraxia	Contralateral to lesion
	Anterior cerebral artery (ACA)	Hemiparesis (leg > face+arm) Incontinence	Contralateral to lesion
Vertebral	**Posterior cerebral artery (PCA)**	Hemianopia Amnesia Thalamic pain Cortical blindness	Nuclear symptoms ipsilateral to lesion, sensory and pyramidal signs contralateral
	Cerebellar Basilar	LOC, Dysphagia Dysarthria Facial weakness Bilateral sensory problems Ataxia Nystagmus Diplopia	

Summary of neurological conditions
Syncope
Arrhythmia-induced syncope
Sudden onset, without aura, patient can appear pale and pulseless before rapid recovery. Patient appears flushed after recovery. Can be due to Stokes–Adams' attack (transient asystole) or ventricular tachycardia (VT).

Cough syncope
Rare – occurs in patients with COPD following a prolonged period of coughing.

Exertional syncope
During exertion due to poor cardiac output secondary to pericardial, myocardial (HOCM) or valvular heart disease (AS).

Head-movement-induced syncope
May have stimulated the carotid sinus in carotid sinus hypersensitivity. Could be caused by extending the neck on gazing upwards and thereby exacerbating vertebrobasilar arterial insufficiency.

Micturition syncope
Uncommon, can occur in males with prostatism who stand to empty their bladders and the decreased bladder wall pressure causes reflex vasodilatation and thereby syncope.

Postural syncope

After prolonged standing, or sudden standing after being seated/lying down. Can be due to dehydration, or poor vasomotor reflexes secondary to autonomic neuropathy.

Vasovagal syncope

Simple faints can be secondary to pain or fear and occur when the patient is standing or occasionally when sitting. Prodrome involves feeling hot, nauseous, weak and light-headed and the patient may appear pale and sweaty. There may be myoclonic jerks but incontinence is rare and recovery is rapid and without amnesia. LOC is due to peripheral vasodilatation and reciprocal hypotension.

UMNL vs. LMNL

In lower motor neuron lesions everything goes down. In **UP**per motor neuron lesions things go **UP**.

Examination

		UMNL	LMNL
I	Inspection	Slight loss muscle mass	Decrease in muscle mass
		Fasciculations	
		Fibrillations	
		Clonus	
Tickle	**T**one	↑ (spastic)	↓ (flaccid)
Patients	**P**ower	↓	↓
Get	**G**ait	Spastic gait Foot drop	
Really	**R**eflexes	↑	↓
		Up-going toe	Normal toe movements
		(also in babies)	
Cool	**C**oordination	N/A	N/A
Smiles	**S**ensation	N/A	N/A

Cerebellar disorders

Examination

I **T**ickle **P**atients **G**et **R**eally **C**ool **S**miles:
  Inspect, Tone, Power, Gait, Reflexes, Coordination, Sensation
I Inspect (**STAN**)
   S Scanning, Slurred, Staccato speech – ask patient to say 'British constitution'

T Tremor (intention)
A Aids for walking such as walking sticks or Zimmer frames
N Nystagmus
T Tone
  Hypotonia
P Power
  N/A
G Gait (**WAR**)
  W Wide-based
  A Ataxia (truncal)
  R Romberg's sign is detected with the patient standing. With feet together ask the patient to close their eyes; if they lose their balance it is a positive Romberg's sign.
R Reflexes
  N/A
C Coordination (**DUFF**)
  D Dysdiadochokinesis
  U Undo and redo a button, they should find this difficult
  F Finger-nose test will show past-pointing – dysmetria
  F Feet, heel-shin test
S Sensation
  N/A

Or (**DANISH GP**)
  D Dysdiadochokinesis – poor rapid alternating movements
  A Ataxia (truncal)
  N Nystagmus
  I Intention tremor
  S Scanning or Slurred speech – ask patient to say 'British constitution'
  H Hypotonia
  G Gait abnormality – exaggerated broad-based
  P Past-pointing – dysmetria

Guillain–Barré syndrome
Features (5 As)
A Acute inflammatory demyelinating polyneuropathy
A Ascending paralysis
A Autonomic neuropathy
A Arrhythmias
A All peripheral neuropathies are distal except Guillain–Barré. Remember all Neuropathies are at the Nail end of the limb except **GB** which Goes closer to the Body. All myopathies are proximal except Myotonic Dystrophy which affects Distant Muscles.

Examination

I Tickle **P**atients **G**et **R**eally **C**ool **S**miles:
Inspect, Tone, Power, Gait, Reflexes, Coordination, Sensation
I Inspect
  Arrhythmias
T Tone
P Power
  Ascending paralysis
G Gait
R Reflexes
C Coordination
S Sensation
  Peripheral neuropathy

Hand nerve palsies

Median nerve palsy (LOAF)

- Carpal tunnel syndrome – median nerve trapped at the wrist

Motor examination is based upon the muscles the median nerve supplies (LOAF):
L Lateral two lumbricals – paper held between digits and try to pull it out
O Opponens pollicis – thumb touches all finger tips
A Abductor pollicis brevis – point finger up towards nose
F Flexor pollicis brevis – bring thumb across to little finger

Sensory examination demonstrates area of paraesthesia on lateral palm and thumb, index, middle and half of the ring finger. Pain may extend to arm and shoulder.
  Complete examination by looking for:
- Tinel's sign
- Phalen's test

Ulnar nerve palsy (MAFFIA)

The ulnar nerve can become impinged at the elbow. *Hand of benediction.*
  Motor examination is based upon the muscles the ulnar nerve supplies (**MAFFIA**):
M Medial two lumbricals – cannot flex 4th and 5th digits at MCP joints
A Adductor pollicis – cannot adduct thumb
F Flexor carpi ulnaris – cannot flex wrist
F Flexor digitorum profundus (FDP)
I Interossei: palmar interossei – AD-duction (PAD)
             dorsal interossei – AB-duction (DAB)
A Abductor digiti minimi

BRANCHES OF THE BRACHIAL PLEXUS

ULNAR NERVE

MOTOR FUNCTION

AB-DUCTION OF
4th AND LITTLE FINGER

MEDIAN NERVE

SENSORY
FUNCTION

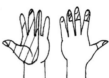

MEDIAN NERVE

MOTOR FUNCTION

OPPOSITION OF THUMB
AND LITTLE FINGER

ULNAR NERVE

SENSORY
FUNCTION

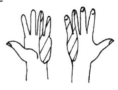

RADIAL NERVE

MOTOR FUNCTION

DORSIFLEXION
OF WRIST

RADIAL NERVE

SENSORY
FUNCTION

FIGURE 9.13

BRANCHES OF THE SCIATIC NERVE

PERONEAL NERVE :-

MOTOR FUNCTION
DORSIFLEXION
OF ANKLE

PERONEAL NERVE :-

SENSORY FUNCTION

DORSAL
SURFACE

TIBIAL NERVE :-

MOTOR FUNCTION

PLANTAR
FLEXION
OF ANKLE

TIBIAL NERVE :-

SENSORY
FUNCTION

PLANTAR
SURFACE

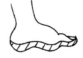

FIGURE 9.14

Sensory examination demonstrates paraesthesia on medial palm and little finger and half ring finger.

Complete examination by looking for Froment's sign:

Froment's sign

Ask the patient to hold a piece of paper between the tip of the thumb and the tip of the index finger and not let you pull it away. If the patient finds this difficult and uses pad-to-pad pinch, this indicates a weak adductor pollicis and the patient is positive for Froment's sign

Radial nerve palsy

The radial nerve can be impinged in the armpit, often by using crutches incorrectly.

Motor examination identifies weakness of the wrist and finger extensors and of the supinator.

Sensory examination reveals a small area of paraesthesia over the anatomical snuff box.

Lambert–Eaton's myasthenic syndrome (LEMS)

Definition

Autoimmune disorder of voltage-gated calcium channels on presynaptic membrane of the neuromuscular junction which prevents the release of acetylcholine and thereby prevents muscle contraction. It needs to be differentiated from myasthenia gravis. *See* LEMS vs. MG, p. 173.

Examination

I Tickle Patients Get Really Cool Smiles:

Inspect, Tone, Power, Gait, Reflexes, Coordination, Sensation

I Inspect (**AIM**):

    A Autonomic symptoms (dry mouth)

    I Impotence (ask about – do not inspect)

    M Muscles of respiration and face not usually affected, if affected not as severe as MG

T Tone

P Power

    Proximal myopathy

G Gait

R Reflexes

    Reduced or absent

C Coordination

S Sensation

Investigation (AIR)

A Antibodies to calcium channels

I Incremental response in repetitive nerve stimulation

R Radiology, CXR for a possible lung malignancy

LEMS vs. MG (SMARM)

		LEMS	*MG*
S	Synapses	Presynaptic auto-Ab	Postsynaptic auto-Ab
M	Myopathy	Proximal	Distal
A	Activity	Improves with activity Symptoms worse in a.m.	Worsens with activity Symptoms worse in p.m.
R	Respiratory and facial muscles	Not usually affected	Affects respiratory and facial muscles
M	Malignancy	50% associated with malignancy (Often small-cell lung ca.)	Associated with thymoma

Motor neurone disease (MND)
Aetiology (CAM)
MND is due to the degeneration of neurons in the Cranial nerve nuclei, Anterior horn cells and Motor cortex. Both UMN and LMN signs are present but there is no sensory involvement. It does not affect the external ocular movements. Three varieties can be distinguished:

Amyotrophic lateral sclerosis (ALS)
Approx. 50% of patients

Progressive muscular atrophy
Approx. 25% of patients

Bulbar palsy
Approx. 25% of patients

Examination
I Tickle Patients Get Really Cool Smiles:
I Inspect (**FAB-W**)
   F Fasciculations of tongue, back, and thigh (LMN)
   A Aspiration pneumonia – secondary to bulbar palsy
   B Bulbar palsy (UMN)
   W Wasting (LMN)
T Tone
   Spasticity (UMN)

P Power
  Weakness (UMN and LMN)
G Gait
  Spastic gait (UMN)
  Foot drop (UMN)
R Reflexes
  Brisk reflexes (UMN)
  Plantars up-going (UMN)
C Coordination
  Not affected
S Sensation
  Not affected

Multiple sclerosis

Definition
Disorder of autoimmune aetiology, leading to demyelination.

Epidemiology (MS)
MS is a feminine title (MS) and this condition is predominantly in females (2:1)

Well-known people with MS
Cellist Jacqueline du Pre, comedian Richard Pryor, television presenter Montel Williams

History
- Bath, unable to get out of a hot bath – Uhthoff's phenomenon
- Impotence in males
- Nystagmus
- Ophthalmoplegia – often the first sign
- Overactive bladder – urinary urgency
- Scanning speech

Examination
I Tickle Patients Get Really Cool Smiles:
  Inspect, Tone, Power, Gait, Reflexes, Coordination, Sensation

Charcot's triad
(Not to be confused with Charcot's triad of cholangitis) **SIN**
S Scanning speech (dysarthria), Syllable durations are equalised
I Intention tremor
N Nystagmus

I Inspect (**SAND**)

S Slurred speech, Scanning speech
A Ataxia
N Nystagmus
D Diplopia, Depression
T Tone
P Power
  Spasticity and weakness
G Gait
  Ataxia
  Wide-based gait
R Reflexes
C Coordination
  Dysdiadochokinesis
  Intention tremor
  Past-pointing
S Sensation
  Lhermitte's phenomenon – electric-shock-like sensations down the back
    and sometimes the thighs on bending the neck
  Neuropathic pain

Or (**DEMYELINATION**):
D Diplopia, Dysmetria, Dysdiadochokinesis, Depression
E Eye movement painful – optic neuritis
M Motor signs – weakness, spasticity
Y nYstagmus
E Elevation in temperature – Uhthoff's phenomenon – classic description
  is 'unable to get out of a hot bath'.
L Lhermitte's phenomenon – electric-shock-like sensations down the back
  and sometimes the thighs on bending the neck
I Intention tremor
N Neuropathic pain – trigeminal neuralgia, dysaesthesia
A Ataxia
T Talking is slurred – dysarthria
I Impotence
O Overactive bladder – urinary urgency
N Numbness – pins and needles (sensory)

Myasthenia gravis
See LEMS vs. MG, p. 173.

Definition
From the Greek for weak muscle and the Latin *gravis* meaning grave. MG
is an autoimmune neuromuscular disease due to autoantibodies to acetylcholine receptors on the postsynaptic neuromuscular junction. This leads
to fatiguability.

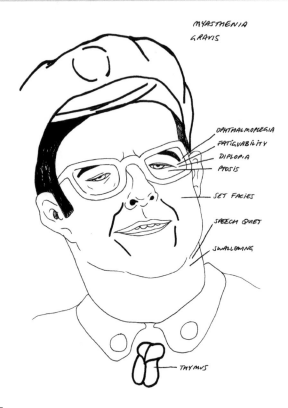

MYASTHENIA
GRAVIS

OPHTHALMOPLEGIA
FATIGUABILITY
DIPLOPIA
PTOSIS

SET FACIES

SPEECH QUIET

SWALLOWING

THYMUS

FIGURE 9.15

Well-known people with MG
Indian actor Amitabh Bachchan, possibly entrepreneur Howard Hughes, entrepreneur Aristotle Onassis

Examination
I **T**ickle **P**atients **G**et **R**eally **C**ool **S**miles:
    Inspect, Tone, Power, Gait, Reflexes, Coordination, Sensation
I Inspect
    S Set facies with poor Smile, and Snarling appearance
    S Sad-looking (**Grave**-looking)
    S Swallowing is poor
    S Speech is quiet
    S Stick or other walking aid due to muscle weakness
T Tone
    Normal
P Power
    Decreased, proximal weakness greater than peripheral. Characterised by FATIGUABILITY.

G Gait
  Normal
R Reflexes
  Decreased
C Coordination/Clonus
  Normal
S Sensation
  Normal
  Myasthenia gravis can be confined to the eyes:
  Diplopia
  Ophthalmoplegia
  Ptosis

The fatiguability is nicely demonstrated in the eyes, ask the patient to keep looking upwards and the ptosis will worsen.

Myotonic dystrophy
Definition
Inherited muscle wasting disorder. The disease shows 'anticipation' where it presents at an earlier age in successive generations.

Famous people with myotonic dystrophy
Possibly the pharaoh Akhenaten

Examination
I Tickle **P**atients **G**et **R**eally **C**ool **S**miles:
  Inspect, Tone, Power, Gait, Reflexes, Coordination, Sensation
I Inspect (**SHAME**):
  S Snarling Smile, Sad-looking, Sagging (drooping) mouth
  H Hair loss, frontal balding and wasting at the temples
  A Apathetic looking
  M Myopathic face – myopathies are usually proximal except myotonic dystrophy (**MD** – **M**yopathy **D**istant)
  E Eyes – ptosis, cataracts, wearing thick glasses
T Tone
  Myotonia (slow relaxation of muscles) – most apparent as difficulty in RELEASING GRIP WHEN SHAKING HANDS (worse in cold conditions).
P Power
  Weak forearms
G Gait
  Normal
R Reflexes
  Decrease

C Coordination/Clonus
  Normal
S Sensation
  Normal

This **A**utosomal dominant condition shows **A**nticipation, it increases in severity with each generation.

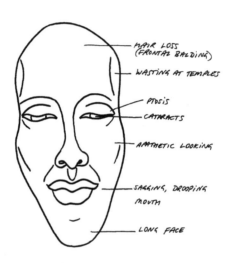

FIGURE 9.16

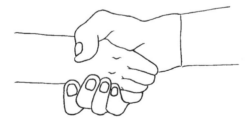

FIGURE 9.17

Parkinson's disease

Definition
Parkinson's disease was originally called the 'shaking palsy' – a movement disorder of the extrapyramidal system.

Famous people with Parkinson's disease
Boxer Muhammad Ali, actor Michael J Fox, General Franco, Adolf Hitler, Chairman Mao, Pope John Paul II, actor Vincent Price, actor Terry Thomas

History (CRAM)
C Cannot get out of a chair or bed easily
R Rolling over in bed at night is difficult
A Activities of daily living hindered – bathing, dressing (buttons and shoelaces in particular)
M Micrographia – handwriting becomes smaller

Examination
I Tickle **P**atients **G**et **R**eally **C**ool **S**miles:
Inspect, Tone, Power, Gait, Reflexes, Coordination, Sensation
I Inspect
    S Stolid, stoic mask-like facies
    S Shaking (resting tremor)
    S Slow movements (bradykinesia)
    S Speech – quiet, slow and monotonous

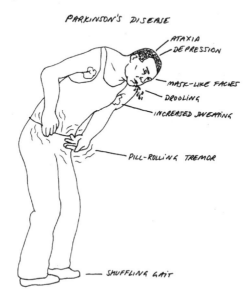

FIGURE 9.18

179

S Slow Sinuous repetitive movements – athetosis

S Seborrhoea – increased oily secretions from Sweat glands of skin

S Sialorrhoea – drooling

T Tone

S Stiffness in muscles – increased tone

P Power

Normal or decreased, from atrophy secondary to lack of movement

G Gait

S Standing up can make them feel dizzy, ataxia (loss of balance)

S Short, Shuffling gait with reduced arm Swinging (festinating gait)

R Reflexes

Normal

S Should be glabellar tap positive

C Coordination

S Small writing – micrographia

S Sensation

S Sensations may be abnormal – paraesthesia

Complications of PD (4 Ds)

D Depression

D Dementia

D Autonomic Dysfunction – postural hypotension, constipation, urinary retention or overflow incontinence, erectile dysfunction

D Death (often pneumonia or PE)

Stroke and TIA

Remember that a stroke affects the cerebrum which is **uppermost** in the brain, the signs are known as **Upper** motor neurone signs, and tone and reflexes are **increased**. *See* UMNL vs. LMNL, p. 168.

Examination

I Tickle Patients Get Really Cool Smiles:

Inspect, Tone, Power, Gait, Reflexes, Coordination, Sensation

I Inspect

S Speech problems – dysphasia/dysarthria

S Stick or other walking aid due to muscle weakness

S Sight is affected – homonymous hemianopia

T Tone

Raised on affected side

Clonus

P Power

Decreased on affected side – hemiparesis. There may be facial weakness

G Gait

Abnormal

R Reflexes

    Increased on affected side

    Babinski present on affected side (up-going plantars) – 'up-going' plantar is not foot retracted due to pain

C Coordination

    Normal or poor if dominant side is affected

S Sensation

    Decreased on affected side

I would complete my examination by examining the cardiovascular system especially, check the pulse for atrial fibrillation, check for heart murmurs, check the blood pressure and for signs of hypertensive heart disease and auscultate for carotid bruits. I would also test the cranial nerves to look for **UP:**

U Upper motor neurone signs on one side

P Pseudobulbar palsy

10

Psychiatry

Contents
- Psychiatric history
- Mental state examination
- List of psychiatric terms
- Cognitive disorders: dementia, delirium, focal brain syndromes (Wernicke's encephalopathy, Korsakoff's syndrome)
- Depressive disorders
- Eating disorders: anorexia nervosa, bulimia nervosa
- Mania and hypomania
- Bipolar affective disorder
- Neurotic disorders: obsessive compulsive disorder (OCD), post-traumatic stress disorder (PTSD)
- Schizophrenia
- Somatic and somatoform disorders: somatisation disorders, hypochondriacal disorder

The psychiatric examination relies heavily upon a detailed history taking which is called diagnostic interviewing. The diagnostic interview can be used to ascertain if the patient's behaviour fits a specific diagnosis under the six major classifications of mental illness.

Psychiatric history
The aim of the history is to give an accurate picture of that patient – 'paint them with words' – to this end it is important to 'quote verbatim' wherever possible. The psychiatric history can take approximately an hour and therefore building a good rapport with the patient is highly important.

Patient's profile
- Full name
- Age

- DoB
- Marital/relationship status
- Occupation
- Racial/ethnic origin
- Religion
- Reason and source of referral
- Opening paragraph (set the scene)

Presenting complaint

Quote verbatim from the patient what they think the main problem is (**NOT SAD**)

N Nature
O Onset
T Treatment (and its outcomes)
S Severity
A Alleviating and Aggravating factors
D Duration and time course

Past psychiatric history

A chronological account of all past psychiatric illness including episodes that were not brought to the attention of doctors or treated. Often psychiatric illness goes unrecognised and untreated.

DIAGNOSIS/SYMPTOMS	DATE	TREATMENT	OUTCOME (ONGOING/RESOLVED)

Treatment mnemonic (TABS) like TABlets

T Treatment
A Adherence/compliance
B Benefits
S Side effects

Past medical history

General enquiries (FAWR)

F Fever
A Appetite
W Weight loss (unintentional)
R Reduced energy/lethargy

Neurology (HEAD)
H Headaches
E Epilepsy/fits/blackouts
A Auditory problems or dizziness
D Dizziness, Double vision

Medications
- Alternative medications (herbal remedies, dietary supplements)
- Drug reactions and allergies
- Medications (psychiatric and non-psychiatric)

Family history
Draw a genogram and follow with at least a paragraph about family dynamics. Any familial psychiatric or mental illness?

Personal history
Birth/infancy (BREAST)
B Birth timing and complications
R bReast fed or bottle fed
E Earliest memory
A Accidents in childhood
S Separation from mother
T Targets met (growth and development)

Childhood (FUNS)
F Family relationships
U Upbringing
N Nursery and early schooling
S Socialising, friends, Sporting and academic achievements

Adolescence (PUBE)
P Peer relationships (including sexual)
U Unusual relationships/behaviours/bullying at school
B Bio-psycho-social pubertal development
E Errors/antisocial behaviours, alcohol or drug misuse

Adulthood (SONS)
S Sexual and marital history (relationships, children)
O Occupational history (jobs, promotions, sacked, satisfaction)
N Network of friends and support
S Seeing into the future, goals and plans

Social history (SAADLERS)
S Smoking in pack years (20/day for 1 year = 1 pack year)

A Alcohol (1 unit = ½ pint lager, 1 glass of wine, 1 measure of spirit females should have less than 14 units/week and males less than 21 units/week)

ADL Activities of Daily Living, including job and accommodation

E Enjoyment activities and hobbies, ask about recreational drugs

R Religious/spiritual affiliations

S Social support, relationships, family and friends

Forensic history (CRIM)

C Chronological account of charges, convictions, sentences for any offences

R Record attitude to their past (regret/blasé/proud)

I Impact it has had on patient and family

M 'Masked' criminal activity (undetected by authorities)

Premorbid personality (CAB)

The patient's personality before the onset of the illness. Personality consists of:

C Cognitions (ways of thinking)

A Affectivity (emotions and feelings)

B Behaviour (interpersonal, reaction, self-control)

Mental state examination

The Mental State Examination (MSE) is used for assessing and recording a patient's state of mind at the time of interview. Mental states change over time and the MSE can be repeated and compared. Write out the headings for the various points of the MSE and annotate them throughout the interview process. A mnemonic for remembering the MSE is:

A	A	Appearance
B	Boring	Behaviour
S	Subject	Speech
M	Matter	Mood and affect
T	This	Thoughts
P	Psychiatry	Perception
C	Claptrap	Cognitive function
I	Is	Insight
R	Really	Risk assessment

Appearance and behaviour (AIM)

A Appearance

I Interactions

M Movements

APPEARANCE	INTERACTIONS	MOVEMENTS
Underweight	Aggressive	Automatism (repetitive unconscious gestures such as lip smacking, chewing, or swallowing)
Overweight	Attentive	
Clean	Cooperative	Ambitendency (tendency to act in opposite ways or directions – the presence of opposing behavioural drives)
Well presented	Defensive	
Dress style	Evasive	
Hair	Facial expressions	Catalepsy (nervous condition, muscular rigidity, fixed posture regardless of external stimuli and decreased sensitivity to pain)
Jewellery	Eye contact	
Emaciated	Excited	
Unshaven	Friendly	Echopraxia (involuntary repetition or imitation of the observed movements of another)
Unkempt	Hostile	
Dishevelled	Indifferent	Limp
Underdressed	Interested	Mimicry
Overdressed	Playful	Posturing
Bizarre	Seductive	Psychomotor agitation (series of unintentional and purposeless motions that stem from mental tension and anxiety)
		Psychomotor retardation (slowing down of thought and a reduction of physical movements)
		Rigidity
		Shuffling
		Somnambulism (sleep-walking)
		Semiconscious
		Hyperactive
		Walk
		Tremor
		Tic (sudden, repetitive, non-rhythmic, stereotyped motor movement or vocalisation involving discrete muscle groups)
		Twitches

Speech

- In the Mental State Examination it is the form of speech that is of interest rather than its content – rate, volume, quality (speed, quantity, accents, clarity)
- Fluency and coherence (reaction, structure, construct)

RATE, VOLUME, QUALITY	FLUENCY AND COHERENCE
Accented	Dysarthria (motor speech disorder)
Emotional	Echolalia (repetition of vocalisations made
Hesitant	by another person)
Lisps (unable to produce certain speech sounds)	Palilalia (repetition or echoing of one's
Loud	own spoken words)
Monotonous	Rehearsed
Mumbled	Responsive
Mutism	Stereotypical
Pressured	Talkative
Rapid	Unspontaneous
Rushed	Verbigerative (wordy)
Responsive	Volubility (fluency)
Slurred	
Stuttered	
Stuttering	
Taciturn (silent)	
Vocal dysphonia (voice impairment)	
Whispered	

Mood and affect

How the patient reports their emotions is called the mood, and how the mood appears to you is the affect. Some emotions are listed below:

Agitated	Expansive
Alexithymic (deficiency in understanding, processing, or describing emotions)	Fearful
	Flat
Ambivalence	Grieving
Angry	Gleeful
Anhedonic (lack of pleasure)	Inappropriate
Anxious	Irritable
Appropriate	Labile
Blunted	Lowered
Depressed	Panicked
Dysphoric (unpleasant mood, the opposite of euphoric)	Restricted
Ecstatic	Tense
Elevated	
Euphoric (sense of elation, usually exaggerated)	
Euthymic (normal, non-depressed, reasonably positive mood)	

Thoughts (content/form)

Divided into content and form

Content

Preoccupations, worries, phobias, recurrent thoughts. Is the thought content normal or abnormal within perceived social and cultural norms; is it an obsession,[3] overvalued idea[4] or delusion[5]?

- Compulsion (repetitive behaviours aimed at reducing anxiety, often seen in OCD)
- Delusion
- Egomania (obsessive preoccupation with one's self)
- Erotomania (delusion in which the affected person believes that another person is in love with him or her)
- Hypochondria (excessive preoccupation about having a serious illness)
- Monomania (obsession with one idea or subject)
- Obsession (often seen in OCD)
- Overvalued idea
- Poverty of thought
- Pseudologia fantastica (person grossly exaggerates symptoms or even lies in order to get medical attention – seen in malingering and Munchausen's syndrome)
- Trend of thought (thinking with a tendency toward or centring on a particular idea with a particular affect)

Form

Describes the flow of thought

- Abstract thinking (thinking characterised by the ability to use concepts and to make and understand generalisations)
- Autistic thinking
- Circumstantiality (disturbed pattern of speech or writing characterised by delay in getting to the point because of the interpolation of unnecessary details and irrelevant parenthetical remarks)
- Clang associations (thought disorder wherein words are chosen or repeated based on similar sounds, instead of semantic meaning, 'He ate the skate')
- Concrete thinking (inability to abstract)
- Condensation (The process by which a single symbol or word is

---

3 **Obsession** – repetitive irrational thoughts that are recognised by the patient to be irrational. Themes are commonly religious, sexual or violent.

4 **Overvalued idea** – unreasonable and sustained preoccupation with a belief that is not quite delusional in intensity, e.g. an anorexic who believes she is fat around the thighs and has to lose weight.

5 **Delusion** – a false belief that is firmly held in spite of evidence to the contrary. It is not in keeping with cultural, religious and social norms.

associated with the emotional content of several, not necessarily related, ideas, feelings, memories, or impulses, especially as expressed in dreams)
- Derailment (thought disorder in which ideas slip off the track on to another which is obliquely related or unrelated)
- Drivelling (to babble)
- Flight of ideas (nearly continuous flow of rapid speech that jumps from topic to topic, with discernible associations, distractions, or plays on words, but in severe cases so rapid as to be disorganised and incoherent – seen in mania and manic episodes of schizophrenia)
- Formal thought disorder or thought disorder (disordered language that is presumed to reflect disordered thinking – usually considered a symptom of psychotic mental illness)
- Glossolalia (speaking in tongues, fluent vocalising, or, less commonly, writing of speech-like syllables, often as part of religious practice)
- Illogical thinking
- Incoherence
- Irrelevant answers
- Loosening of associations (manifestation of a severe thought disorder characterised by the lack of an obvious connection between one thought or phrase and the next)
- Neologism (new words – may only have meaning to the person using them)
- Perseveration (uncontrollable repetition of a particular response, such as a word, phrase, or gesture, despite the absence or cessation of the original stimulus – usually seen in organic disorders of brain, head injury, delirium or dementia, but can be seen in schizophrenia)
- Tangentiality (pattern of speech characterised by oblique, digressive, or irrelevant replies to questions)
- Thought block (abrupt and complete interruption in the stream of thought, strongly suggestive of schizophrenia)
- Transitory thinking (thinking characterised by derailments, substitutions and omissions)
- Word salad/schizophasia (confused and often repetitious language, a symptom of formal thought disorder, seen in psychoses)

Perceptions (HID)
H Hallucinations (a false perception in the absence of a real external stimulus)
I Illusions (a false perception of a real external stimulus)
D Dissociation (the mind separates a person's thoughts, memories, actions from their normal consciousness – can be as dissociative amnesia,[6]

---

6 **Dissociative amnesia** – inability to remember important personal information to a degree that cannot be explained by normal forgetfulness. Often occurs as a result of a traumatic incident.

depersonalisation[7] or derealisation[8])

Cognitive function

Cognitive state can fluctuate and needs to be measured. A variety of tools have been developed to this end including the Abbreviated Mental Test Score (AMTS) which is a 10-point test mainly validated in the elderly (*see* elderly medicine chapter, p. 63). The Mini Mental State Examination (MMSE) is a 30-point test used to screen and estimate the severity of cognitive impairment. It can be repeated to chart the course of cognitive changes in individuals over time.

See Mini mental state examination (MMSE), p. 67.

Insight (FAB)

F Feel they need treatment?
A Abnormal experiences recognised as abnormal?
B Believe they have a psychiatric disorder?

Risk assessment (ASH)

A Act
S State
H History

A Act (ROPE)
    R Realised a method
    O Outcome and intent
    P Planning/Precautions against being found
    E Evidence of similar acts
S State (current mental state) (HARM):
    H Habitus/attitude
    A Affect
    R Risk to others
    M Mental disorders
H History (HIS):
    H History (psychiatric/medical/family)
    I Individual triggers (recent life events)
    S Social circumstances

---

7 **Depersonalisation** – a sense of detachment from the self. Feel like a robot or watching themselves from the outside. Depersonalisation disorder may also involve feelings of numbness.

8 **Derealisation** – objects in an environment appear altered to an individual. It is often accompanied by depersonalisation. Normal things may seem strange, unreal, distant, or two-dimensional.

Cognitive disorders

In severe cognitive impairment a collateral history may be required. Dementia can be differentiated from delirium because consciousness is not clouded.

Dementia (5 As)

A Amnesia
A Aphasia
A Apraxia
A Agnosia
A Arithmetic (inability to perform)

Delirium (C DIPPS – DIPPing of Consciousness)

A, and two or more from B

A C   Clouding of consciousness and disorientation
B D   Disorientation or impaired memory
  I   Incoherent speech
  P   Perceptual disturbances such as hallucinations/illusions
  P   Psychomotor changes, either retardation or restless overactivity
  S   Sleep is affected, with insomnia and daytime sleeping

Focal brain syndromes
Wernicke's encephalopathy

Features (A SOAP)

A Altered consciousness (confusion)
S Subacute brain syndrome
O Ophthalmoplegia
A Ataxia of gait/Alcoholics commonly affected
P Prodromal nausea may be present

Korsakoff's syndrome

Features (6 Cs)

C Cognitive impairment revealed when acute state clears
C Cognitive functioning preserved
C Clouding of consciousness does not occur
C Can not lay down new memories, but long-term memory is preserved
C Commonly found in alcoholics due to thiamine deficiency
C Confabulation (makes up answers)

Depressive disorders

The patient has at least two of the core symptoms plus two other symptoms for a minimum duration of two weeks with sustained dysfunction. The more severe the depression the more somatic symptoms and the greater the impact they have on his/her life.

Symptoms (MARDIE)

M Mood is lowered
A Anhedonia
R Reduction of energy
D Decreased concentration
I Ideas of guilt or worthlessness
E Esteem and self-confidence is reduced

Somatic symptoms (LESS)

L Lose appetite, lose weight
E Early morning waking, feel worse in the morning
S Sleep is poor
S Sex drive is lost

Suicide risk factors (SAD PERSONS)

S Sex (male)
A Age (older)
D Depression
P Previous attempt
E Excessive alcohol or substance abuse
R Rational thinking is lost
S Sickness (chronic illness)
O Organised plan
N No social supports
S Stated intention to self-harm

Eating disorders: anorexia nervosa and bulimia nervosa

An eating disorder is a psychological compulsion to eat or avoid eating that has a negative impact on both physical and mental health. The two main eating disorders in psychiatry are anorexia nervosa and bulimia nervosa.

Famous people with anorexia nervosa

Singer Karen Carpenter, actress Calista Flockhart, actress Audrey Hepburn, author Franz Kafka, actress Mary-Kate Olsen

Anorexia nervosa (FLAB)

F Fear of Flab and Fatness
L Loss of weight is deliberate (BMI below 17.5)
A Appetite suppressants, diuretics, restricted intake of calories, excessive exercise, induced vomiting and purgation to lose weight
B Bodily function is disturbed due to endocrine and metabolic changes.

Famous people with bulimia nervosa

Singer Paula Abdul, actress Jane Fonda, singer Geri Halliwell, singer/

songwriter Elton John, Diana, Princess of Wales

Bulimia nervosa (PURGE)

P Pattern of overeating (binge) followed by **P**urge with **P**urgatives or vomiting
U Urea and electrolytes can be disturbed and physical complications
R Repeated bouts of overeating
G Get depressed
E Earlier episode of anorexia nervosa is common

Mania and hypomania
Mania (INSPIRED – because patients often have inspired creativity)

I Increased energy
N Need for sleep is decreased
S Symptoms for 7 days with sustained dysfunction
P Pressure of speech
I Insight is lost
R Reduced inhibitions
E Expansive grandiose ideas and Elevated mood
D Decreased concentration and irritability

Hypomania (HYPO has four letters)

Hypomania is a less severe presentation of mania. Symptoms have to be present for **four days** with only mild/moderate dysfunction, insight tends to preserved.

Bipolar affective disorder
Famous people with bipolar affective disorder

Musician Kurt Cobain, actress Carrie Fisher, author Stephen Fry, artist Vincent van Gogh

    Bipolar affective disorder is a disorder characterised by changing mood/ activity that swings between mania and depression.

Neurotic disorders

Neurotic disorders include obsessive-compulsive disorder and post-traumatic stress disorder.

Famous people with obsessive–compulsive disorder

Actor Leonardo DiCaprio, actress Cameron Diaz, entrepreneur Howard Hughes, actor Billy Bob Thornton, entrepreneur Donald Trump

Obsessive compulsive disorder (TIRED)

T Thoughts are obsessional and recurrent and can be unpleasant or obscene

I Impulses can be embarrassing

R Resistance to compulsions makes anxiety worse

E Events that may seem unlikely have to be prevented with rituals and stereotyped behaviours

D Doubts and constant rechecking of items such as locks, gas and electricity

Post-traumatic stress disorder (PTSD)

P Protracted response to a stressful event

T Trauma is relived in repeated episodes (flashbacks or nightmares)

S State of autonomic hyperarousal with hypervigilance and insomnia

D Depression and suicidal ideation

Schizophrenia

Definition

Schizophrenia ('splitting of the mind') is a disease involving distortions of thinking and perception. In order to make diagnosis the patient must have had at least one of the 'first-rank features or two of the other features, for a period of at least one month.

Famous people with schizophrenia

Nobel Laureate in Economics, John Forbes Nash Jr. (of *A Beautiful Mind* fame), author Jack Kerouac

Positive symptoms

Sometimes called Type I schizophrenic symptoms

(**THREAD** – they lose the **THREAD** of reality)

T Thought phenomena (echo, insertion, withdrawal, broadcasting)

H Hallucinations may occur, usually auditory

R Reduced contact with reality, break in the train of thought

E Emotional control may be disturbed with inappropriate laughter or anger (incongruous affect)

A Arousal may lead to worsening of symptoms

D Delusions may occur (Delusional perception, Delusions of control, influence or passivity)

Negative symptoms

Sometimes called Type II schizophrenic symptoms

LESS (patient appears **LESS** active)

L Loss of volition, apathy and social withdrawal

E Emotional flatness, blunt affect

S Speech is poor, monosyllabic if at all

S Slowness in thought and movement, psychomotor retardation may occur

Somatic and somatoform disorders

These disorders are characterised by multiple physical symptoms such as pain, nausea, depression, dizziness.

Somatisation disorders (SOMA)

S Symptoms may be referred to any part of the body
O Ongoing for at least two years
M Multiple, recurrent and frequently changing, medically unexplained symptoms
A Associated with disruption of social, interpersonal, and family behaviour

Hypochondriacal disorder (PAP)

P Persistently preoccupied with the possibility of having a serious physical disorder
A Appearances or sensations which are normal are interpreted as abnormal and distressing
P Persistent preoccupation with somatic complaints or physical appearance (dysmorphia)

11

Respiratory system

Contents

- Respiratory history
- Respiratory examination: pre-examination checklist, inspection, (general, hands, face, neck and JVP and trachea, chest movements), palpation, percussion, auscultation, inspection, abdomen and legs
- The six major symptoms of respiratory disease
- Breath sounds
- Causes of hyperventilation
- Cough
- Percussion note

Respiratory history

Refer to general examination

Respiratory examination

Pre-examination checklist (WIPERS)
Inspection

General (ABC)

A Appearance (PANTS)

- **P**ursed lip exhalation? (helps increase intrabronchial pressure above that of the surrounding alveoli thereby preventing collapse of bronchioles)
- **A**ccessory muscle use? (cervical muscles – sternomastoids, scalene and trapezii lift the thoracic cage and aid inspiration)
- **N**asal flaring?
- **T**ired? (may require non-invasive ventilatory support)
- **S**itting forward and holding onto support? (fixes the shoulder girdle and allows latissimus dorsi to aid expiration)

B **B**ehaviour

- Comfortable at rest? Respiratory rate (RR) approximately 14/min is normal.
- Depth of respiration – air hunger (Kussmaul's breathing)? Cheyne–Stokes' breathing – alternating apnoea with hyperventilation?
- Mode of breathing – thoracic or diaphragmatic? Most women use their intercostal muscles more than their diaphragms, males are the opposite.
- Paradoxical chest movement? (Fractured ribs?)

C Connections – oxygen, nebuliser, non-invasive ventilation, ventilator, inhalers, cigarettes or nicotine supplements, sputum cup (check the contents)

Hands (CASH) or (TEACH CAST)
C Clubbing
A Asterixis
S Small-muscle wasting
H Hypertrophic pulmonary osteoarthropathy (HPOA). Causes pain and swelling in the hands, wrists, feet and ankles and X-rays show subperiosteal new bone formation.

Or
T Tobacco staining
E Erythema
A Asterixis

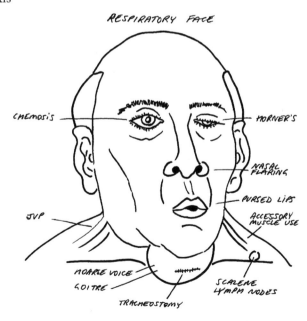

FIGURE 11.1

C Clubbing
H Hypertrophic pulmonary osteoarthropathy (HPOA)
C Cyanosis
A Anaemia
S Small muscle wasting
T Tremor

Face
- Anaemia – pallor conjunctivae
- Chemosis (CO_2 retention, the tear drop that does not fall), Cushingoid face? From long-term steroid use? Constricted pupil, could be part of Horner's syndrome see MATES. Central cyanosis, look under the tongue and at the lips
- Cough – productive (LRTI), dry cough (ACEi, asthma), bovine cough (paralysed vocal chords)
- Horner's syndrome – apical lung cancer (ptosis, miosis, anhidrosis)
- Inflamed tonsils (URTI)
- Nasal obstruction – deviated septum, nasal polyps (asthma), swollen turbinates, sinusitis, (examine the nose with a torch)
- Teeth – tar staining, rotten (can lead to LRTI or lung abscess)
- Tongue – leucoplakia (smoking, spirits, sepsis, sore teeth, syphilis)
- Voice – hoarse (recurrent laryngeal nerve palsy)

Neck and JVP and trachea
- Accessory muscles of inspiration are hypertrophied
- Goitre (tracheal impingement)
- JVP – significant if it is more than 3 cm
- Lymph nodes, **especially the scalene nodes.** Roll your fingers behind the clavicles. Instruct the patient to cough or to bear down. Nodes which are >0.5 cm in diameter, round and firm are often pathological,

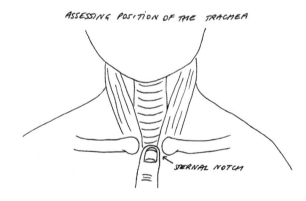

ASSESSING POSITION OF THE TRACHEA

STERNAL NOTCH

FIGURE 11.2

commonly from metastases from a bronchial carcinoma. Hard, craggy nodes may be healed calcified TB.

- Obese neck with receding chin (sleep apnoea)
- Scars (tracheostomy)
- Trachea – advise the patient that this might be uncomfortable; place middle finger in the sternal notch, and the ring and index finger on either side. If deviated it could be due to an upper lobe problem. Remember the trachea is PUSHED by Pleural effusion and tension Pneumothorax and CARRIED OFF by Collapse and Fibrosis.

Chest movements (HAS AIR)
H **H**yperventilation or hypoventilation, **H**arrison's sulcus – depression above costal margin (rickets, childhood asthma)

A **A**bnormal skeleton – pigeon chest/pectus carinatum (rickets), funnel chest/pectus excavatum (congenital defect), kyphosis, scoliosis, lordosis, kyphoscoliosis

S **S**cars – indicative of previous surgery

A **A**nteroposterior diameter increased (barrel chest)

I **I**ntercostal/subcostal recession – airways obstruction

R **R**ibs broken? Chest drain?

Palpation
Before palpating ask the patient if they are tender in any place and examine that last

Chest expansion
Usual expansion is 4–5 cm check that it is bilateral.

Symmetrical reduction of chest wall expansion
Overinflated lungs   Bronchial asthma, emphysema

Stiff lungs   Diffuse pulmonary fibrosis (each inspiration may halt abruptly – 'doorstep' breathing)

Unilateral reduction of chest wall expansion
Absent expansion   Empyema and pleural effusion

Reduced expansion   Pulmonary consolidation and collapse

Percussion
Vocal fremitus – use the ulnar edge of the hand in between the intercostal spaces. Ask the patient to repeat the phrase 'ninety-nine'. Increased sensation indicates consolidation or absent over areas of effusion or collapse.

Auscultation
Ask the patient to 'Breathe in and out through your mouth, keeping your

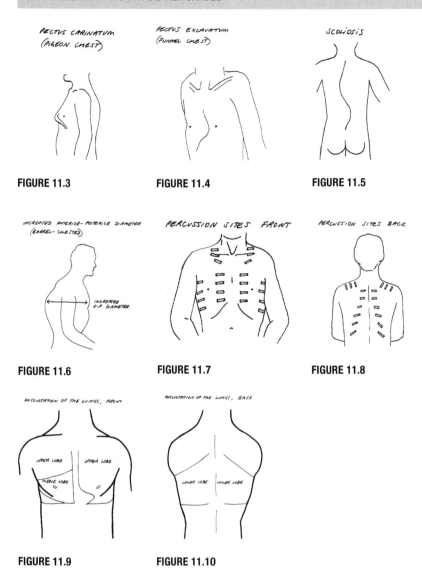

PECTVS CARINATVM
(PIGEON CHEST)

PECTVS EXCAVATVM
(FUNNEL CHEST)

SCOLIOSIS

FIGURE 11.3

FIGURE 11.4

FIGURE 11.5

INCREASED ANTERIOR-POSTERIOR DIAMETER
(BARREL-CHESTED)

INCREASED
A-P DIAMETER.

PERCUSSION SITES FRONT

PERCUSSION SITES BACK

FIGURE 11.6

FIGURE 11.7

FIGURE 11.8

AUSCULTATION OF THE LUNGS, FRONT

UPPER LOBE

UPPER LOBE

MIDDLE LOBE

AUSCULTATION OF THE LUNGS, BACK

LOWER LOBE

LOWER LOBE

FIGURE 11.9

FIGURE 11.10

mouth open, nice deep breaths please.' Auscultate the posterior chest. Avoid auscultation within 2–3 cm of the midline.

Vocal resonance – ask the patient to repeat the phrase 'ninety-nine' while you listen to the chest with a stethoscope. There is muffled vocal resonance over normal lung, increased vocal resonance if there is consolidation, decreased or absent vocal resonance if there is effusion or collapse. **Whispering pectoriloquy** is where whispered speech is clearly heard. There is an increased transmission of high frequencies and speech has a bleating quality, **aeogophony** – goat voice. *See* Breath sounds, p. 203.

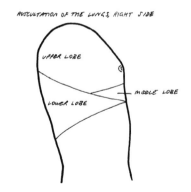

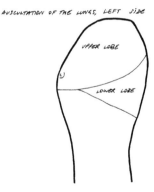

FIGURE 11.11   **FIGURE 11.12**

Heart
- Auscultate the heart

Inspection
- Pemberton's sign (SVC obstruction)

Ask the patient to raise their arms over their head – Pemberton's sign is positive if the patient develops a plethoric complexion, non-pulsatile JVP elevation and inspiratory stridor

Abdomen and legs
- Abdominal breathing

Assess the legs for swollen calves (DVT), presence of surgical stockings (preventing DVT), peripheral cyanosis and peripheral oedema (congestive heart failure).

The 6 major symptoms of respiratory disease
Cough
Most common symptom in respiratory disease. Caused by stimulation of sensory nerves of the mucosa in pharynx, larynx, trachea or bronchi.
See Cough, p. 204.

Chest pain
Chest pain is divided anatomically into central (retrosternal) and lateral. Lateral chest pain can be further divided into pleural and chest wall. Musculoskeletal pain can be central but not retrosternal.

CENTRAL / RETROSTERNAL	LATERAL (PLEURAL)	LATERAL (CHEST WALL)
Acute mediastinitis	Pneumonia*	Fractured rib*
Cardiac chest pain*	Malignancy	Invasion of rib by tumour/metastases
Lesions of great vessels	Pulmonary embolism	
Mediastinal tumours	TB	Herpes zoster
Mediastinal emphysema		Spinal nerve impingement due to vertebral disease
Oesophageal disorders		
(GORD)		Coxsackie B infection (Bornholm disease)
Tracheitis		
*most common		

Haemoptysis

Haemoptysis needs to be differentiated from haematemesis by a careful history. Regular frank haemoptysis or blood streaking over a week suggests bronchial carcinoma, however recurrent episodes over a duration of years with purulent sputum indicates bronchiectasis.

Common causes of haemoptysis:
- Abscess (lung)
- Bronchial carcinoma
- Embolism (pulmonary)
- TB
- Less common causes of haemoptysis:
- Aspergilloma
- Bronchitis (acute and COPD)
- Mitral stenosis

Shortness of breath (dyspnoea)

Due to any or all of the following:

Ventilatory drive is increased. This can be due to hyperventilation secondary to stimulation of the respiratory centre or an increase in physiological dead space due to ventilation-perfusion (VQ) mismatch. Causes of VQ mismatch include collapse, consolidation, PE and pulmonary oedema. These trigger a response of increased respiratory rate and also increased depth of ventilation.

See Causes of hyperventilation, p. 204.

Work of breathing is increased. This can be due to airflow obstruction (bronchial asthma, COPD), decreased pulmonary compliance (pulmonary fibrosis, pulmonary oedema) and restricted chest expansion (kyphoscoliosis, ankylosing spondylitis and respiratory muscle paralysis).

Respiratory muscle function is impaired. Caused by neuromuscular disorders affecting the intercostal muscles and diaphragm (Guillain–Barré, polio, muscular dystrophies and myasthenia gravis). Increased respiratory rate and the sensation of breathlessness are not necessarily related. In severe hypoxaemia the sensation of breathlessness is triggered. Hypercapnia induces hyperventilation and breathlessness in otherwise normal individuals but those with chronic type II respiratory disease may be less responsive to this stimulus.

Sputum

TYPES OF SPUTUM	APPEARANCE	CAUSE
Mucoid	Grey, white, clear	COPD, chronic asthma
Mucopurulent/ purulent	Yellow, green, brown	Bronchopulmonary bacterial infection
Rusty	Rusty	Pneumococcal pneumonia
Serous	Clear, may be frothy or pink	Acute pulmonary oedema

Wheeze
Musical sounds produced by narrowed bronchi. Can be inspiratory or expiratory but more like to be expiratory. Stridor is NOT a wheeze, it is caused by the partial obstruction of a major airway (larynx) and needs to be investigated urgently. Stridor is more pronounced on inspiration.

Breath sounds
- **Normal breath sounds** – vesicular
- **Wheeze/rhonchi** – sounds produced by air passing through narrowed bronchi (asthma), often described as 'musical'
- **Stridor** is harsh sound on Inspiration due to partial obstruction of a major airway.
- **Aegophony speech** (bleating goat) – indicates consolidation
- **Crepitations/crackles** – heard on inspiration due to the reopening of occluded small airways (pulmonary oedema/fibrosing alveolitis)
- **Pleural rub** – creaking sound due to movement of stiff pleural surfaces, e.g. pleurisy secondary to pneumonia
- **Bronchial breathing** – indicates lung tissue has lost its usual spongy texture and has become firm secondary to consolidation or fibrosis. Sounds similar to movement of air through the larynx. High-frequency bronchial breathing indicates consolidation (lobar or segmental pneumonia). Low-frequency bronchial breathing indicates fibrotic lung tissue. Bronchial breathing is present if four criteria are met:
  1 Both inspiratory and expiratory breath sounds are blowing in nature (tubular).
  2 The expiratory sound is of equal duration and loudness in comparison to the inspiratory sound and of high pitch.

3 There is a pause between the end of inspiration and the beginning of expiration.

4 Vocal resonance is increased and therefore whispering pectoriloquy is heard. A whisper can be clearly heard through the stethoscope indicating extreme consolidation.

Causes of hyperventilation

- Anxiety/exertion leading to central arousal
- CO_2, increased arterial $PaCO_2$, respiratory acidosis
- H, increased arterial H^+ concentration, metabolic acidosis (Kussmaul's breathing)
- O_2, decreased arterial PaO_2, detected in aortic, carotid and brainstem chemoreceptors due to pneumonia, anaemia, shock
- Pulmonary J receptor activation secondary to pulmonary oedema

Cough

ANATOMY	COMMON AETIOLOGY	TYPE OF COUGH
Pharynx	Postnasal drip	Persistent
Larynx	Laryngitis, croup, whooping cough	Harsh 'barking' sound +/- stridor
Trachea	Tracheitis	Painful
Bronchi	Asthma	Dry/productive, worse night
	Bronchial ca.	Persistent +/- haemoptysis
	Bronchitis (acute or COPD)	Dry/productive, worse mornings
	Bronchiectasis	Productive, and postural changes increase sputum production
	Pneumonia	Dry, later productive
Pulmonary oedema		Pink frothy sputum especially at night
Left recurrent laryngeal nerve palsy	Lung ca.	Bovine cough

Percussion note

The percussion note becomes impaired or dull when normal air-filled lung is separated from the chest wall by pleural fluid/thickening or when the lung loses its air due to consolidation, collapse or fibrosis.

Resonant Normal lung

Impaired Pulmonary consolidation/collapse/fibrosis, liver

Dull Pulmonary consolidation/collapse/fibrosis, liver

Stony dull Indicates fluid – pleural effusion

Tympanic Hollow viscus – pneumothorax, bowel

Hyperresonant Pneumothorax, emphysematous lung. It may prove difficult to differentiate hyperresonant from resonant or tympanic.

12

Rheumatology

Contents
- Rheumatoid history
- Rheumatoid examination: pre-examination checklist, inspection (general)
- Rheumatological examination of the hands
- Ankylosing spondylitis
- Rheumatoid arthritis
- Scleroderma
- CREST syndrome
- Rheumatoid hand

Rheumatoid history
Joint pain – distribution, duration, onset, periodicity (morning stiffness RA, ankylosing spondylitis), severity

Associated features – disability, family history, non-articular symptoms, previous medical history, previous treatment

The normal joint
There are three general types of joint where two or more bones come together, each type is characterised by different degrees of movement and function:
- **Cartilaginous** – intervertebral joints, pubic symphysis, joint between the first rib and manubrium
- **Fibrous** – cranial sutures, inferior tibiofibular joint
- **Synovial** joints (all other joints) – cartilage-coated articular surfaces, surrounded by a fibrous capsule lined by an epithelial layer of synovium. The synovial joint is characterised by the largest degree of movement and the most important pathologically.

Rheumatoid examination
Pre-examination checklist (WIPERS)
The rheumatology examination follows the pattern of look, feel and touch.

Inspection (look)
General
A **A**ppearance – observation of the patient walking should allow the assessment of any gait abnormalities, butterfly rash (SLE), steroidal appearance (cushingoid – RA)
B **B**ehaviour – comfortable at rest, leaning forward
C **C**onnections – aids for walking, sticks, crutches, frame, wheelchair, oxygen, nebuliser, cigarettes or nicotine supplements, sputum cup (check the contents), cardiac monitor, ECG leads, drug cardex, observation chart contains vital signs such as temperature, BP, pulse, respiratory rate, oxygen saturations, GCS, MEWS/PARS score

The most common rheumatological examination is of the hands. Place the sitting patient's hands on a pillow, palms down. Examine each joint in term moving from tips (peripherally) to more centrally. Observe the pattern of joint involvement, associated skin conditions, muscle wasting, deformities. Particular features to identify are:
- Inflammation
- Instability
- Points of tenderness
- Range of movement
- Swelling

Rheumatological examination of the hands
Nails (SPORT)
- **S**plinter haemorrhages (SLE, RA)
- **P**in-sized pitting (**p**soriatic arthritis)
- **O**nycholysis – nail separation from the distal bed (psoriatic arthritis)
- **R**idges (psoriatic arthritis)
- **T**hickening – hyperkeratosis (psoriatic arthritis)

Fingers and wrist
- Anaemia
- Arthritis mutilans (shortened fingers)
- Calcinosis (scleroderma) and Contraction deformity of the fingers (scleroderma)
- Deformities – Swan neck and boutonnière (both RA)
- Entrapment of ulnar nerve
- Muscle wasting on the dorsum of the hand (RA)

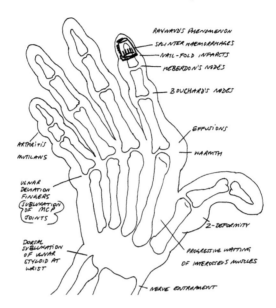

FIGURE 12.1

- **N**odes – Bouchard's nodes (PIP – OA)/Heberden's nodes (DIP – 1st MCP – OA)
- **R**edness (inflammation)
- **S**ausage-shaped digits (psoriatic arthritis)
- **T**elangiectasia (scleroderma)
- **U**lnar deviation of the fingers (MCP – RA)
- **Z** deformity of thumb (RA)

Palm (WASTE)

W Wasting
A Anaemia
S Scars from operations
T Tightening of the skin
E Erythema

Palpation (feel) NEWTS

Fingers (patient's hand should be palm down):
- Nodules (RA)
- Effusions
- Warmth
- Tenderness
- Swelling

Movement (touch)

Carefully palpate and try to move each joint systematically, with both thumbs

- Assess active movements and then passive movements

Normal movements:
- Dorsiflexion   (normal is 75 degrees)
- Palmar flexion   (normal is 75 degrees)
- AB-duction   (normal is 75 degrees)
- AD-duction   (normal is 75 degrees)

Special tests (STOP TAP)

S Strength of grip (patient squeezes examiner's fingers)

T Tinel's sign (carpal tunnel) – tap on the patient's flexor retinaculum, Tinel's positive with paraesthesia over median nerve distribution

O Opposition test – hold the thumb and little finger together

P Paper grip – patient holds a piece of paper between thumb and index fingertips; whilst holding can they open their other fingers

T Trigger finger (RA)

A Activities of daily living – the patient writes their name with a pen or undoes a button

P Palmar tendon crepitus (tenosynovitis) – place the pads of your finger tips on the patients palm whilst they flex and extend their MCPs, listen for crepitus during motion and also palpate for thickened tendons and nodules

DO NOT do the volar subluxation test, inexperience may lead to damage

The volar subluxation test

Hold the proximal phalanx between thumb and forefinger, move the MCP joint, normal joints will have little movement

Head

- Acuity decreases (seronegatives)
- Dry mouth (Sjögren's)
- Ears – tophi (RA)
- Elbows – tophi (RA)
- Eyes can not completely close on command (scleroderma)
- Eyes – dry eyes (Sjögren's)/red painful eyes (seronegatives), scleritis (RA nodule in eye)
- Hair – lupus hair (short, broken – SLE)
- Rash – butterfly (SLE)
- Salt and pepper pigmentation and Stretched (face-lift) face (SLE)

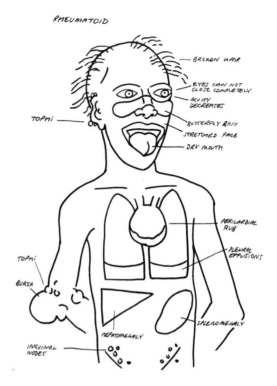

FIGURE 12.2

Chest (PEC)
P Pericardial rub (RA, SLE)
E Effusions in the lungs, fibrosis (RA, SLE)
C Chest wall has thickened skin (scleroderma)

Abdomen (HIPS)
H Hepatomegaly (SLE)
I Inguinal nodes (RA)
P Psoriasis in lumbosacral area (psoriasis)
S Splenomegaly (RA, SLE)

Elbows
- Bursa
- Effusions (joint swelling)
- Epicondyle tenderness (lateral – tennis elbow)/(medial – golfer's elbow)
- Nodules – hard (RA), firm (gout)
- Psoriasis
- Warmth

Shoulders
- Movements, active and then passive
- AB-duction   (normal is 150°)
- AD-duction   (normal is 50°)
- Flexion   (normal is 180°)
- Extension   (normal is 60°)
- External rotation   (normal is 60°)
- Internal rotation   (normal is 90°)

TMJ
- Examination of parotid (Sjögren's)
- Grating or other noises
- Swelling
- Tenderness (RA)

Neck and spine
- Exaggerated kyphosis (ankylosing spondylitis)
- Head tilt (RA – atlantoaxial subluxation)
- Loss of lumbar lordosis (ankylosing spondylitis)
- Pressure over sacroiliac joints elicits pain, bilateral (ankylosing spondylitis/Reiter's), unilateral (Reiter's)
- Spasms over vertebrae

Special tests
Schober's test
Ask the patient to stand, mark the 5th lumbar spine and also 10 cm above that mark, ask the patient to flex their waist (lean forward) and the mark should increase to >15 cm.

Ankles and feet
Inspection:
- Arches are flattened
- Calluses on deformed joints (RA)
- Clawing of the toes
- Crowded toes (RA)
- Foot drop (RA)
- Hallux valgus (lateral deviation of the big toe)
- Oedema, ankle – (steroid use)
- Swelling
- Tophi (gout)
- Ulcerations (Felty's)

Palpation
- Achilles tendonitis (Ankylosing spondylitis), Achilles tendon nodules (RA)
- Seronegatives – plantar fasciitis
- Squeeze all metatarsophalangeal joints together for tenderness (RA)
- Peripheral neuropathy (spinal cord compression)
- Warmth

Movements of the foot
- Dorsiflexion   (normal is 20 degrees)
- Plantar flexion   (normal is 50 degrees)
- Eversion
- Inversion
- Individual toe movements

Ankylosing spondylitis
Ankylosing spondylitis derives its name from the Greek *ankylos* (bent) *spondylos* (vertebrae). A seronegative spondyloarthritis, a chronic, progressive inflammatory arthritis affecting joints in the spine and the sacroilium causing fusion of the spine.

Famous people with ankylosing spondylitis
Sportsman Michael Atherton, sportsman Michael Slater, presenter Ed Sullivan

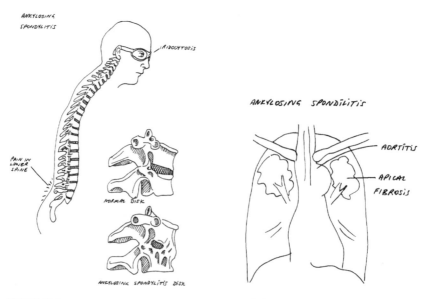

FIGURE 12.3   **FIGURE 12.4**

History and examination (YOGA HIPS)

Y **Y**oung people are affected (18–30) males : females 3:1
O **O**nycholysis
G **G**eneralised fatigue
A **A**ortitis/**A**pical lung fibrosis
H **H**LA-B27 (90%), CRP and ESR raised during acute exacerbations
I **I**ridocyclitis – eye pain and photophobia
P **P**ain in lower spine/physical activity improves the pain
S **S**chober's test positive
   X-ray – bamboo spine

Rheumatoid arthritis

Famous people with rheumatoid arthritis

Actress Lucille Ball, heart transplant pioneer Christiaan Barnard, actress Kathleen Turner, artist Renoir

- Boutonnière deformity involving the PIPs
- Dorsal subluxation of ulnar styloid at the wrist
- Enlargement of the MCP
- Interosseous muscles progressively waste
- Rupture of the 4th and 5th extensor tendons when there is also inflammation within extensor tendon sheaths
- Swan-neck deformity involving the DIPs
- Ulnar deviation at the MCP
- Z-thumb deformity

Extra-articular features

- Mostly associated with vasculitis:
- Atlantoaxial subluxation
- Haematology (anaemia), Hepatic (Felty's syndrome)
- Inflammation (diffuse), involving lungs, pericardium, pleura, sclera
- Nail-bed infarcts
- Ocular – episcleritis, keratoconjunctivitis sicca
- Peripheral neuropathy
- Raynaud's phenomenon
- Splinter haemorrhages

Scleroderma

Definition

A multi-system disorder characterised by fibrosis and degenerative changes in the skin and many internal organs. Clinical manifestation of scleroderma.

SCLERODERMA

S **S**kin – hyperpigmentation, telangiectasia, subcutaneous calcification, fingertip ulcers, sclerodactyly

Index

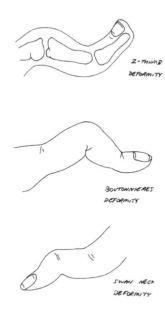

Z - THUMB DEFORMITY

BOUTONNIERES DEFORMITY

SWAN NECK DEFORMITY

FIGURE 12.5

BOUTONNIERES DEFORMITY
PIP JOINT POKES THROUGH THE EXTENSOR
EXPANSION FOLLOWING RUPTURE OF ITS
CENTRAL POSITION

SWAN NECK DEFORMITY
FIBROTIC CONTRACTURE OF
INTEROSSEUS AND LUMBRICAL MUSCLES.

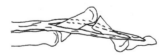

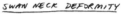

FIGURE 12.6   **FIGURE 12.7**

C Cardiac – myocardial fibrosis, cardiac failure
L Lung – Interstitial lung disease, aspiration pneumonia, pulmonary hypertension
E oEsophageal dysfunction
R Raynaud's phenomenon
O Obstruction (pseudo) of intestine
D Dry eyes/ mouth
E Endocrine (hypothyroidism)
R Renal failure leading to malignant hypertension
M Microstomia, perioral furrowing, pursed lip, Myopathy
A Arthritis

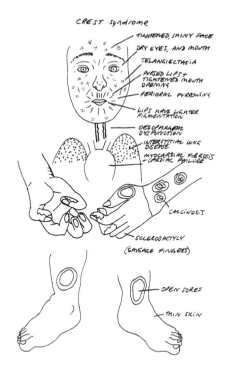

CREST syndrome

TIGHTENED, SHINY FACE
DRY EYES, AND MOUTH
TELANGIECTASIA
PURSED LIPS +
TIGHTENED MOUTH
OPENING
PERIORAL PURROWING
LIPS HAVE LIGHTER
PIGMENTATION
OESOPHAGEAL
DYSFUNCTION
INTERSTITIAL LUNG
DISEASE
MYOCARDIAL FIBROSIS
+ CARDIAC FAILURE
CALCINOSIS
SCLERODACTYLY
(SAUSAGE FINGERS)
OPEN SORES
THIN SKIN

FIGURE 12.8

CREST syndrome (CREST POT)

CREST syndrome is a limited form of scleroderma associated with antinuclear and anticentromere antibodies. A systemic inflammatory rheumatic disease:

C Calcinosis
R Raynaud's syndrome
E oEsophageal dysmotility
S Sclerodactyly
T Telangiectasia
P Pulmonary artery hypertension (can lead to heart failure)
O Open leg sores leading to chronic infections (badly healing)
T Thin skin

A quote from the always quotable William Osler:

> *He who studies medicine without books sails an uncharted sea, but he who studies medicine without patients does not go to sea at all.*

Happy sailing!

Index